D1071142

A Parent's Guide to
HEART
DISORDERS

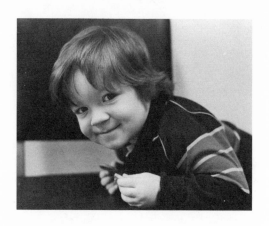

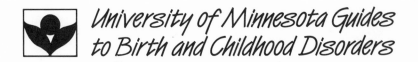
University of Minnesota Guides to Birth and Childhood Disorders

Subjects of Forthcoming Volumes

Cerebral palsy
Cleft lip and palate
Cystic fibrosis

Kidney disorders
Leukemia
Sickle-cell anemia and
   thalassemia

Spina bifida
Spine deformities

A Parent's Guide to HEART DISORDERS

James H. Moller, M.D., professor of pediatrics and Paul F. Dwan Professor of Pediatric Cardiology, University of Minnesota

William A. Neal, M.D., professor and chairman of pediatric cardiology, West Virginia University School of Medicine

and

William R. Hoffman, science writer

618.92
Mol

University of Minnesota Press, Minneapolis

Published by the University of Minnesota Press, 2037 University Avenue Southeast, Minneapolis, MN 55414. Published simultaneously in Canada by Fitzhenry & Whiteside Limited, Markham. Printed in the United States of America.

Library of Congress Cataloging-in-Publication Data

Moller, James H., 1933-
   A parent's guide to heart disorders.
   (University of Minnesota guides to birth and childhood disorders)
      Bibliography: p.
      Includes index.
      1. Pediatric cardiology—Popular works. I. Neal, William A., 1940-   . II. Hoffman, William R.
III. Title. IV. Series. [DNLM: 1. Heart Diseases—in adolescence. 2. Heart Diseases—in infancy & childhood. WS 290 M726p]
RJ421.M566 1987   618.92'12   87-19225
ISBN 0-8166-1478-4

CONTENTS

FOREWORD

A Parent's Guide to Heart Disorders is the first book of a series in which we hope to address the needs not only of parents but also of physicians and persons concerned with the care of children with relatively common disorders. We used as a model *The Child with Down's Syndrome*, written by David W. Smith, M.D., and Ann Asper Wilson and first published in 1973 by W. B. Saunders, Philadelphia. The book is very valuable because it makes the complex concepts of genetics and pediatrics understandable to parents. Such is the goal of our series.

In *A Parent's Guide to Heart Disorders*, the authors discuss how the heart functions and the methods for determining whether it is working properly. The more common congenital and acquired disorders as well as abnormalities of heartbeat are covered in lucid terms. Because all cardiac anomalies could not be mentioned in the text, an appendix of the rarer conditions has been provided. Such important questions as how to select a heart surgeon, when to seek a second opinion, and what to expect during the usual hospital stay for investigative tests and for surgical procedures are also addressed. No less important are the authors' helpful suggestions on dealing with the myriad problems of the infant and school-age child with a cardiac problem. Last, the authors discuss prevention of heart disease, and the hope that recent research has provided. This book is meant to help parents cope; by understanding, their fears may, at least in part, be alleviated.

This book was written by James H. Moller, M.D., William A. Neal, M.D., and William R. Hoffman. Dr. Moller is a professor of pediatrics and the Paul F. Dwan Professor of Pediatric Cardiology,

School of Medicine, University of Minnesota. He is currently chief of staff at the University of Minnesota Hospital. He has written eight textbooks and over one hundred other publications on various aspects of pediatric cardiology and has served on and directed an inordinate number of committees: community, university, and national-professional. He represents that wonderful amalgam of tender concern and professional excellence. Dr. Neal received his graduate training in pediatrics and pediatric cardiology at the University of Minnesota, under the aegis of Dr. Moller. He is now professor and chairman of pediatric cardiology at West Virginia University School of Medicine. He has several dozen publications on pediatric cardiology to his credit, including *Heart Diseases in Infancy*, published by Appleton-Century-Crofts, New York, which he coauthored with Dr. Moller. The doctors were assisted by William Hoffman, a free-lance writer and editor. Mr. Hoffman's educational background, which includes a master of arts degree in journalism and mass communication, has led him to writing and editing in the sciences. As this book illustrates, he has a talent for shaping highly technical material into an understandable, readable whole.

The need for this series is obvious. Parents of a child with a serious disability need answers. They need to know not only the nature of their child's disorder but also its possible causes, its prognosis, the limitations it will impose on the child, the impact it will have on the entire family, and the chances of it recurring in either the parents' future children or in the affected child's children. It is also important that parents be informed about community resources that can help them deal with the disorder. And, certainly, they need to know what they themselves can do to help.

In spite of good intentions, the health professional has not always been an effective communicator. These books are designed to open the lines of communication between the health professional and parents by increasing parents' understanding and providing them with a basic vocabulary for easier and more accurate expression of the worries, doubts, and uncertainties attendant to each disorder. It is our intention that health professionals play a vital part by supplementing each text with their own expertise. We cannot hope to answer all the questions that may be posed by parents, but we believe that each book will go a long way in answering many of the common ones.

R. J. G.

Preface

Nothing is as symbolic of life as a beating heart. The English physician who discovered how the circulatory system works said that the heart is the sun of the bodily universe, just as the sun is the heart of the solar system. The heartbeat is the life pulse.

That is probably why it was so alarming for you when you learned that your infant or child has a heart problem. It is difficult to be prepared for this kind of thing. Your first reaction may have been one of panic. Later, you may have felt trapped, overwhelmed by the emotional, physical, and financial demands of caring for your child and making decisions that could affect his or her survival. You may be uncomfortable in a hospital or clinical environment; the instruments of medical technology can appear threatening.

As pediatricians who specialize in the care of infants and children with heart disease, the two of us have seen many such reactions from parents in our combined 35 years in the field. We devote a part of each day to meeting with parents, discussing their child's heart condition, and recommending the diagnostic and treatment plan we feel is most appropriate.

The outlook for infants and children with heart disease is far better today than it was just a few decades ago. Advances in medicine mean that most children can be treated successfully. The recovery of a seriously ill infant or child is our greatest reward. Time and again we are awed by the recuperative powers of the young. We are also impressed by the inner strength, self-sacrifice, and binding love of their parents. Now and then we share in parents' sorrow and grief over the loss of their child.

Like other fields of medicine, pediatric cardiology is becoming increasingly technical and seemingly removed from society at large. Several years ago, while collaborating on the preparation of a scientific book, we discovered a mutual desire to relate our experiences and knowledge in a book specifically designed for parents of children with heart disease. We perceived a great need for it. Its origin lies in the many questions that parents have asked us about their child's health and treatment.

Over the years we have noticed that informed parents are much better able to allay their child's fears and anxieties about visiting the doctor's office or the hospital. They know how to prepare their child for catheterization and surgery, if such procedures are needed, and to assist in the recovery. The experiences of some of the parents we have worked with are recounted in several chapters in this book.

We have included five appendixes. The first one explains the duties and responsibilities of the medical and hospital staff, the second focuses on quality of care and patient rights, the third discusses congenital heart diseases not covered in chapter 4, the fourth provides a list of addresses for affiliates of the American Heart Association and comparable organizations in Canada and Great Britain, and the fifth is a brief guide to prevention of heart disease. We have also compiled a reading list and a glossary.

We hope this book will answer some of your questions and provide the kind of information that will enable you to understand the nature of your child's heart problem, the types of diagnostic tests used, the experience of surgery, and the special problems you may encounter in raising your child. We also hope you will be reassured and comforted when you read about others who share your experiences.

A Parent's
Guide to
HEART
DISORDERS

Chapter 1
A REMARKABLE PUMP

Before you can understand what is wrong with your child's heart, you must know something about normal heart function and normal murmurs, which are discussed at the beginning of chapter 2. The heart is a relatively simple organ compared with others, so grasping how it works is not as hard as it might seem.

The heart is a pump. It is not an ordinary pump. No other pump could work one hundred thousand times a day and more than two billion times over an average human life span without regular servicing. For sheer durability, the heart is easily the most powerful muscle in the body. Each day it pumps about 4,300 gallons of blood, four times as much blood as gasoline pumped by a typical service station in a given day. Over a lifetime, that is enough blood to fill a small lake.

The ancient Greeks, who gave Western medicine its start, thought the heart was a boiler. For them, the heart was the source of "vital heat," rather than a pump. They also thought the heart was the seat of emotion, an idea with real staying-power in romance. (Consider Valentine's Day.)

Some two thousand years after the Greeks, the English physician William Harvey discovered that the heart beats to circulate blood. In *An Anatomical Treatise on the Motion of the Heart and Blood in Animals* (1628), he wrote: "I begin to think within myself whether it [the blood] might have a sort of motion, as it were, in a circle." With this discovery, Harvey laid the foundation of modern medicine.

The heart pumps blood through blood vessels to various organs in the body. Blood provides oxygen and essential nutrients to the organs and tissues. They need oxygen to keep running, and when blood flows through them, oxygen is removed. The pumping action of the heart creates pressure in the blood vessels, which enables blood to be delivered throughout the body.

The heart is the center of the circulatory system. This system is made up of a large and intricate network of blood vessels running throughout the body from the head to the toes. The heart is located beneath the breastbone. It is about the size of a fist and weighs about four pounds in adults. The heart in a baby is small, compared with an adult's heart. (Think of the difference in size between your fist and your child's fist.)

The heart is a compact organ with four chambers. Two are located on the right side of the heart and the other two are on the left side. The chambers on the right side are called the right atrium and right ventricle (fig. 1). Those on the left side are called the left atrium and left ventricle. The atria receive blood when it returns to the heart. The ventricles, with their thick-muscled walls, are primarily responsible for pumping blood from the heart. The atria are sometimes called the upper chambers and the ventricles the lower chambers.

The heart also has four valves (fig. 2). Two are on the right side and two on the left side. They are one-way valves (blood can flow through them in only one direction). This helps keep blood moving forward through the heart.

How Circulation Works

As you may know, not all blood is the same color. Blood that is rich in oxygen is red. Blood that has passed through an organ, such as the liver, brain, or muscles, from which oxygen has been removed is blue. Blood that returns to the heart from most of the body's organs is blue because it contains carbon dioxide, the exhaust of the cells. This blue blood returns through two large blood vessels (fig. 3). One, called the superior vena cava, drains the head, the arms, and the upper part of the body. The other, the inferior vena cava, drains the lower extremities, including the abdomen. These major veins connect to the right atrium.

The blood in the right atrium passes across one of the four one-

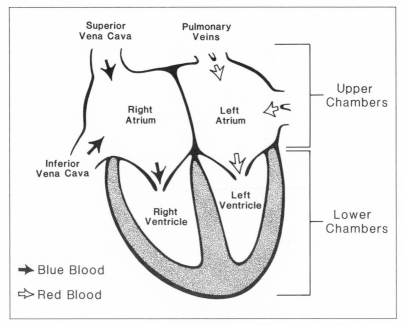

FIGURE 1

Normal heart. The heart has four chambers. The upper chambers are called atria and the lower chambers ventricles. The heart has two sides, right side and left side. Thus, the chambers are labeled right and left respectively. The blue or venous blood returns to the right atrium through the inferior and superior venae cavae and passes into the right ventricle. The red, or oxygenated blood, returns to the left atrium through the pulmonary veins and passes into the left ventricle.

way heart valves, the tricuspid valve, into the right ventricle. This valve has three parts—thin, flaplike structures called leaflets. The tricuspid valve is forced shut when the right ventricle contracts. Thus, the blood that has entered the right ventricle cannot escape back into the right atrium. While it contracts, the right ventricle propels blood out its other opening, the pulmonary valve, forcing it into the pulmonary artery, a large blood vessel that leads to the lungs. The one-way pulmonary valve does not allow blood to pass from the pulmonary artery back into the right ventricle. The blood in the pulmonary artery then flows through a network of blood vessels into both the right and left lungs (fig. 4).

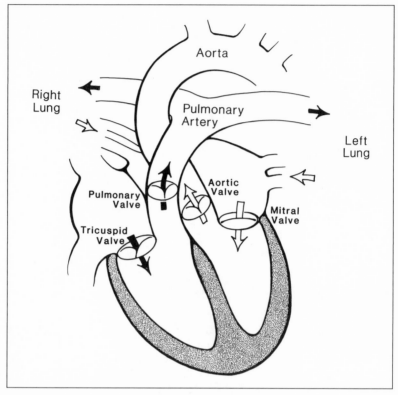

FIGURE 2

Heart valves. The heart has four valves. Two are located on the right side of the heart and two on the left side of the heart. They are one-way valves, permitting blood to flow forward but preventing its return. On the right side of the heart, the tricuspid valve separates the right atrium from the right ventricle, and the pulmonary valve separates the right ventricle from the pulmonary artery, which is the major blood vessel going from the heart to the lungs. On the left side of the heart, the mitral valve separates the left atrium from the left ventricle, and the aortic valve separates the left ventricle from the aorta, which is the major blood vessel that leaves the heart and carries blood to the body.

The blood in the pulmonary artery is blue because it lacks oxygen. When you breathe, oxygen is drawn into the lungs where blood flowing through the lungs picks it up and changes its color from

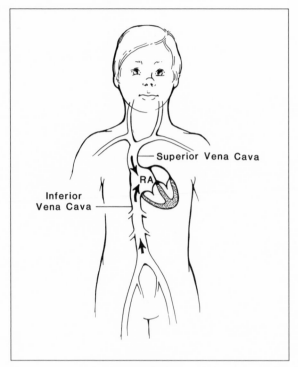

FIGURE 3

Venae cavae. The venae cavae transport blood to the right atrium (RA). The superior vena cava carries blood from the head and arms and the inferior vena cava from the legs and abdomen.

blue to red. This red, oxygen-rich blood returns to the heart through blood vessels called pulmonary veins. There are four pulmonary veins. Two stem from the right lung and two from the left lung. They are attached to the left atrium.

The blood in the left atrium, the upper chamber on the left, passes through the one-way mitral valve into the left ventricle. The mitral valve resembles the tricuspid valve but has only two leaflets. When the left ventricle contracts (the left and right ventricles contract at the same time), the mitral valve closes, forcing blood into the aorta. The aorta is the major artery that carries blood to all the body's organs except the lungs. The aorta is comparable to the pulmonary artery because both carry blood from the heart. At the junction of the

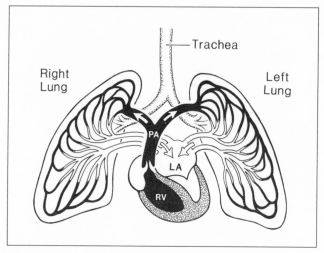

FIGURE 4
Blood circulation through the lungs. The oxygen-poor (blue) blood is
pumped from the right ventricle (RV) to the pulmonary artery (PA). The
PA is the major blood vessel that carries blood from the heart to the lungs.
Within the lungs the PA divides into smaller and smaller blood vessels that
run throughout the right and the left lung. In the lungs the blood comes
in contact with the air that has reached them through the major airway (tra-
chea). Blood returns through pulmonary veins into the left atrium (LA).
This blood is oxygen-rich (red). The oxygen-rich blood is carried through
the left side of the heart and is ejected into the aorta and thus to the body.

left ventricle and the aorta is the one-way aortic valve. It permits
blood to flow from the left ventricle into the aorta, but not in the opposite direction.

As a result of this process of blood passing through each of the
four cardiac chambers and valves, oxygen-rich blood is delivered
into the aorta and from there throughout the body via a multitude
of vessels.

There are three major categories of blood vessels: arteries, which
take blood from the heart and send it to the tissues; capillaries,
which are tiny vessels passing through the tissues in which nutrients, oxygen, and waste products are exchanged; and veins, which
return blood to the heart. The system of blood vessels is like a tree,
with the trunk representing the aorta, the arteries the branches, and
the capillaries the twigs.

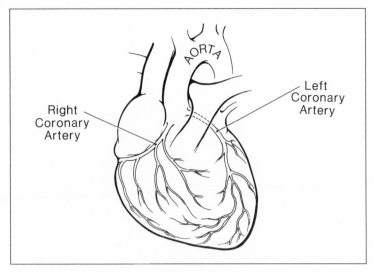

FIGURE 5

Coronary circulation. Two coronary arteries, the right and the left, arise from the root of the aorta. These arteries supply the heart muscle with blood.

Just as body tissues need nutrients and oxygen, so does the heart. The heart receives its nourishment through two small arteries that originate from the aorta just beyond the aortic valve. These are called the coronary arteries (fig. 5). They extend over the surface of the heart and then through smaller and smaller arteries until the blood reaches capillaries that provide nourishment for the heart muscle. Although diseases of coronary arteries are uncommon in children, they are a major cause of cardiac disease in adults.

Checking Your Pulse

Each time your heart contracts, you can feel the pulse beat. You can check your pulse by feeling your wrist for the contraction of the ventricle when it is transmitted by way of the peripheral blood vessels. The normal pulse rate in an adult is about seventy-two times a minute, which indicates that the heart contracts seventy-two times a

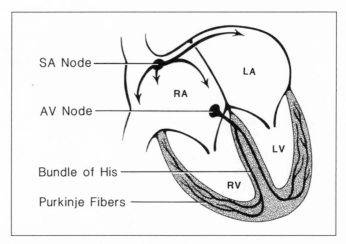

FIGURE 6

Conduction system. The heart has an electrical system through which impulses flow to cause the heart to contract. The major pacemaker is the SA node. This bit of tissue controls the frequency at which the heart beats. Small fibers carry impulses over the right atrium (RA) and left atrium (LA). These impulses converge into a second piece of specialized tissue, the AV node. From there the impulse travels down the bundle of His and into the Purkinje fibers over the ventricular surfaces. This impulse then causes the right ventricle (RV) and the left ventricle (LV) to contract.

minute. When you are exercising, excited, or under stress, your heart contracts at a faster rate, so your pulse rate is faster. The pulse rate is faster in infants and children than in adults (about 100–120 times per minute).

A complex electrical system runs through the two atria and into the ventricles of the heart. This electrical system, a natural pacemaker, is responsible for synchronizing the contraction of the cardiac chambers. It is controlled by the nervous system and chemicals, such as adrenaline, which circulate in the bloodstream. When you exercise or are excited, these chemical messages are released by the brain and your heart rate speeds up. At other times – during sleep, for example – the heart rate slows down. Thus, the pulse rate varies depending on what you are doing.

To maintain orderly contraction, the heart's electrical system is regulated by unique cells that make up what is called specialized conduction tissue. This tissue, shown in figure 6, resembles an electrical system that runs throughout the heart. The parts of the tissue function in an integrated fashion, like an electrical circuit.

The speed and regularity of heartbeats are controlled by a small nodule of tissue in the roof of the right atrium. This tissue, called the sinoatrial or sinus (SA) node, is regulated by nerves that in turn are stimulated by chemicals circulating through the bloodstream. The SA node fires about seventy-two times per minute when you are at rest, producing a heart contraction or pulse each time. It fires faster when you are excited, frightened, or exercising. An electrical impulse is generated by the SA node when it fires, spreading through the pathways in the atria and causing them to contract.

These impulses converge in another small nodule, the atrioventricular (AV) node, located where the atria join the ventricles. The impulse slowly passes through the AV node, allowing time for the atrium to contract to fill the ventricles with blood. The impulse then spreads into the ventricles, causing the whole ventricular wall to contract at once.

This orderly sequence is important—first the atria contracting to fill the ventricles, then the ventricles contracting and emptying. Like a spaceship or a jumbo jet, the heart has multiple safeguards and backup systems. If one part of the conduction system malfunctions, the rest of the system takes over and stimulates the heart.

Chapter 2
THE HEART MAY
BE A PROBLEM

If you are worried that your child might have a heart problem, you should make an appointment with your doctor as soon as possible. The presence of a heart problem can be identified by discovery of a heart murmur, an abnormal sound your doctor may hear when listening to your child's heart. Most murmurs in children do not indicate a heart problem, and these normal murmurs must be distinguished from those that do.

Most heart diseases have fairly clear symptoms and can be recognized more easily than many other diseases. If your child does in fact have a heart disease, he or she may have congestive heart failure, cyanosis, or a serious murmur reflecting a cardiac anomaly (see chapters 4, 5, 6, and appendix C).

Normal Murmurs

"Your child has a murmur." Such a remark can understandably alarm parents, regardless of how it is said. The fact is, though, that most murmurs neither indicate the presence of heart disease nor point to a problem with the circulatory system.

Most heart murmurs are called functional, innocent, or, as we prefer, normal. This means that the heart is normal. Many children have such murmurs. As a safeguard, physicians carefully evaluate a normal murmur just to make sure that it does not indicate an underlying heart problem.

A healthy heart makes only two sounds each time it beats. These sounds are short and are often described as sounding like lub-dub. Thus, when a doctor listens to your heart he or she hears a regular lub-dub, lub-dub, lub-dub. The period between the lub and dub and the dub and lub is silent. The murmur of a crowd suggests noise—background noise, not necessarily loud noise. The murmur of a heart is a long noise occurring between the normal heart sounds of lub-dub.

In all children, at some time, a murmur may be heard. Murmurs are common, particularly in the early school years, but they can be heard in adolescents and, less frequently, in newborn infants. They are more common when the child is excited or has a fever.

In school-age children, the ratio of normal murmurs to significant murmurs is about ninety-nine to one. That is, for every one hundred children in whom a doctor finds a murmur, only one will have a heart problem. Thus the odds are very much in your child's favor. In newborns, the odds are about twelve to one that a murmur is normal, although the overall frequency of murmurs is less in newborns than in school-age children.

If your doctor discovers a murmur, he or she will listen carefully to determine whether it is normal or serious. In school-age children, normal murmurs have particular features that enable doctors to make the correct diagnosis. These features may include the location of the murmur or its loudness and are usually quite different from those of murmurs that indicate the presence of heart disease. The features are usually so typical that no further diagnostic studies, such as electrocardiogram, chest X-ray, or echocardiogram, are required.

In newborns it is more difficult to distinguish between a normal and a serious murmur, and misdiagnosis of a serious murmur as normal may have greater consequences. The physician will look for blue color and breathing or feeding difficulties. Often, additional studies, such as a chest X-ray, are performed. If the X-ray is normal, the odds favor a normal murmur, but your physician may want to see your baby when he or she is two weeks old to determine whether the murmur has persisted.

If your newborn with a murmur has symptoms (fast breathing or feeding difficulty) or an enlarged heart, a cardiac problem is usually present. Your doctor will probably refer you to a cardiologist for further evaluation.

Because an infant or child with a normal murmur actually has a healthy heart, the same care is required as for other children, nothing more, nothing less. He or she requires the same periodic routine examinations that all children require. No special check-ups for participation in sports or physical education are needed. Nor are special laboratory studies needed. Your child should be allowed to engage in a full range of activities, bar none. No special treatment is required for respiratory or other infections.

If your child has a normal murmur, you should relay this information on particular occasions, such as in emergency rooms or whenever your child is examined by a different doctor. Such information may help the physician with his or her evaluation.

In general, doctors do not favor informing the school about normal murmurs. They fear that normal murmurs may be misinterpreted as indicating the presence of a heart problem, which can lead to unnecessary restriction from physical activities. Your school-age child should be reassured that his or her heart is normal. Answer questions directly and honestly.

When you are filling out health forms for school or camps, we advise that you write normal. If there is a place to indicate a murmur under the section on the heart, leave it blank. Your child's heart *is* normal.

Please note that a normal, functional heart murmur will not make your child prone to heart disease in adulthood. Your child's chances for a happy, healthy life are just as great as for a child without a murmur.

Congestive Heart Failure

Congestive heart failure is not a disease in itself but can result from different forms of heart disease. Heart failure does not mean heart attack or heart stoppage. Congestive heart failure is an inability of the heart to do its normal work. It occurs when too great a burden is placed on the heart. The heart is unable to handle its normal workload, that is, to pump blood normally. As a result, blood and fluid back up, usually in both the lungs and the heart.

Nearly 80 percent of all instances of congestive heart failure in children occur in infants less than one year old who have a congenital heart defect. Older children with acquired heart disease make up the rest.

Congestive heart failure is usually easy to diagnose. Four major features are typically present: (1) tachycardia, or an abnormally fast heart rate, which is one way for the heart to compensate for sluggish circulation; (2) tachypnea, or rapid breathing, which indicates congestion in the lungs; (3) hepatomegaly, or an enlarged liver, which denotes congestion in the body; and (4) cardiomegaly, or an enlarged heart, which reflects the decreased ability of the heart to do its work.

The presence of these features enables the physician to make the diagnosis of congestive heart failure. Most children with this problem will be treated in the hospital. Treatment consists mainly of medication. Further diagnostic studies, often including cardiac catheterization, are performed to determine the type of heart problem that caused the failure. Then the underlying condition itself usually can be treated by medications that increase the pumping action of the heart, expand the blood vessels, and help eliminate excess water. Corrective surgery is also an option for children with congestive heart failure.

Cyanosis

Cyanosis is a bluish discoloration caused by a lack of oxygen. Certain congenital heart conditions or lung problems are often responsible. In these cases the blueness is generally present over all the body and is usually worse when the child exercises or exerts himself or herself.

This type of cyanosis should not be confused with the cyanosis present in a lot of normal children, particularly when they are exposed to cold. Healthy children may develop blueness around the mouth or in the fingertips or feet. With activity or warming, this cyanosis disappears.

Chest Pain and Other Symptoms

Chest pain is a symptom that is commonly associated in peoples' minds with heart disease, but it rarely reflects heart disease in children.

The typical chest pain of an adult experiencing a heart attack is described as a crushing or constricting sensation in the center of the chest beneath the breastbone. Usually it lasts for several minutes. Children, on the other hand, may have chest pain unrelated to the heart. Usually this pain, which may originate in the rib cage, is of no medical concern. Also, adults with heart problems often feel tired and listless. These symptoms result from the heart being unable to pump blood adequately. In a child, such fatigue due to a heart problem is uncommon. In fact, most affected children are very active. When tiredness and fatigue exist, their cause is probably something other than a heart problem.

People with severe heart problems may be limited in their abilities to exert themselves physically, and thus may have to stop and rest as they climb stairs or walk. These symptoms are present in adults with heart failure. But most heart problems in children do not limit their ability to exercise, although some children may not be able to exercise at the maximum level. Ordinarily these children are capable of carrying out normal activities in school and at home.

Evaluating the Patient

Under ordinary circumstances, your child's pediatrician or family physician will arrange a referral to a pediatric cardiologist, a specialist in treating heart disease in infants and children, when a heart problem is obvious or suspected.

The cardiologist has a variety of methods available to determine the type of cardiac disease your child may have. Not all these methods are used in each case. Those that provide the necessary information about your child in particular will be selected. In addition to providing clues about the diagnosis, these methods can be used to determine the severity of the condition. This is key information because the type and urgency of treatment may depend on it.

The first thing the cardiologist does is to review the parts of your child's history that may be related to the suspected heart problem. He or she may read the notes or referral letter from the referring physician and ask you a series of questions: When was cyanosis or a murmur first detected? What symptoms, if any, are present? Is your child growing normally? You should answer these questions as completely as possible. Your answers help the cardiologist determine the type and severity of the condition.

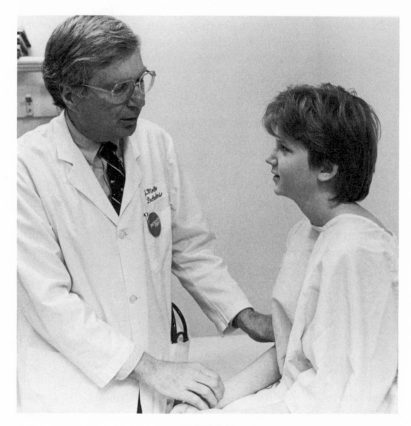

FIGURE 7
Examination. The physician is taking the pulse of this adolescent with
heart disease.

After obtaining the medical history of your child, the physician
will do an examination (fig. 7). Your infant or child is placed on an
examining table, or, in the case of a toddler, seated in your lap for
the examination. He or she will not be as frightened in this position.

It is important for your child to be as quiet as possible during the
examination. A fussy child should be comforted, not scolded.
Efforts to restrain an active or frightened child often backfire. Patience, reassurance, and a positive attitude by both you and the
physician are usually the most successful ways to allay your child's
anxieties and fears.

Physical examination consists of observing the overall state of your child's health and checking for a serious heart murmur or symptoms of cyanosis or congestive heart failure. The cardiologist concentrates on the heart and blood vessels. He or she carefully notes the intensity of the pulse in your child's arms and legs. Unless they have been measured previously, the blood pressures in an arm and leg are read. The cardiologist will then listen to your child's chest, paying attention to the lungs and especially to the heart. Listening to the heart as intently as is necessary often takes several minutes. This should not alarm you. There are several subtle features of the heart that take time to analyze. If your child is restless or if his or her heart is beating very fast, this part of the examination may take longer. The cardiologist may hear the characteristic lub-dub of a healthy heart or the sound of a murmur, which in some ways resembles the purring of a cat. This phase of the examination is crucial for making an accurate diagnosis.

The cardiologist usually examines the abdomen as well, checking the size of the liver and the spleen. As we noted before, the liver is sometimes enlarged (hepatomegaly) in patients with congestive heart failure, and patients with a heart infection may have an enlarged spleen.

Upon completion of the history and physical examination, the cardiologist often has a reasonably good idea whether a problem exists. He or she will usually order a chest X-ray and an electrocardiogram to assist in the evaluation of your child's heart. These studies not only help the cardiologist arrive at an accurate diagnosis but also help to indicate the severity of the defect. It is not always necessary to repeat these tests if they have been done recently, so parents should obtain copies of X-rays, electrocardiograms, and other relevant studies for the cardiologist if they have been done at another clinic. Reports of the studies rather than the studies themselves are usually not sufficient.

If the cardiologist feels that more tests are necessary, they will be scheduled after discussion with you. Ask questions so that you understand the cardiologist's recommendations for additional tests and what the tests entail.

Diagnostic procedures are broadly classified as either *noninvasive* (chest X-ray, electrocardiogram [EKG], echocardiogram) or *invasive* (if an instrument is actually inserted into the body [cardiac catheterization]). Noninvasive procedures are generally associated with little or no risk to your child. Nevertheless, some of these tests are ex-

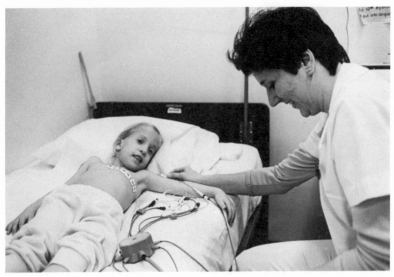

FIGURE 8

Electrocardiogram (EKG). The young girl is lying on a bed with electrodes attached to her arms, legs, and placed across her chest. The technician is recording with a machine from these leads.

pensive and time-consuming and will not be scheduled unless there is sufficient reason. (For a discussion of cardiac catheterization, see chapter 3.)

Electrocardiography

Electrocardiogram, usually called EKG or ECG, is familiar to many people because it is commonly performed in adults. In this technique, small metal plates are attached to both arms and both legs, and a small suction cup is moved to various positions on the chest (fig. 8). The plates and suction cup are attached with wires to a recording device that writes on a special paper, forming a wave pattern as shown in figure 9.

The electrocardiogram furnishes the physician several types of information. It is very useful in detecting irregularities of the heart-

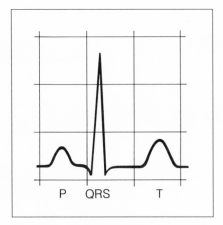

FIGURE 9

Normal electrocardiographic tracing. The impulses of the conduction system cause particular wave forms. The P wave causes contraction of the atrium and the QRS complex, which causes the contraction of the ventricle and the T wave. The T wave represents the heart's return to a neutral electrical status.

beat and in determining the precise type of irregularity. A particular application of this technique is in intensive care units where the electrocardiogram waveforms are continuously viewed on an oscillographic screen while the electrocardiogram is being performed.

The electrocardiogram test is also used to detect enlargement or thickening of heart chambers. Heart disease can alter the circulation and place abnormal stresses on the heart chambers, which cause them to dilate or results in a thickening of the wall. This provides valuable clues to your doctor. The electrocardiogram is also altered by abnormalities of the blood salts or by diseases that affect the heart muscle.

Chest X-ray

Chest X-rays are a very useful diagnostic technique for cardiologists. To obtain satisfactory films, your infant will be placed in a plastic device or strapped to a board to keep him or her stationary.

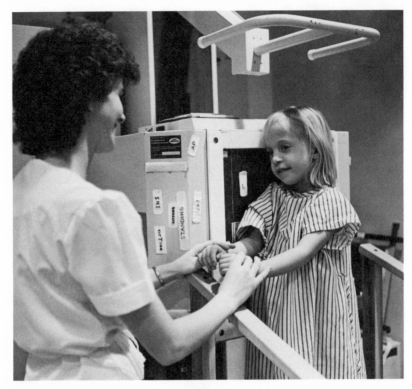

FIGURE 10

Chest x-ray. The girl is standing with her right shoulder to the x-ray screen. The technician is holding the girl's arms out in front of her.

Your infant may cry during the X-ray. This should be expected because he or she probably does not like being restrained. In fact, better X-rays are sometimes obtained when children are crying, because their lungs are expanded. If your child is older, he or she will most likely cooperate for the films. To obtain them, your child may be asked to swallow a pastelike substance containing barium. This material helps outline certain structures of the heart and major blood vessels.

X-rays give the cardiologist information about the overall size of the heart and that of various compartments. It allows the cardiologist to assess the status of blood flow through the lungs, which is

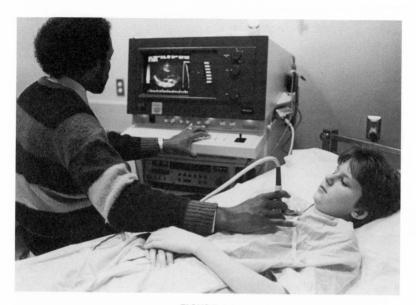

FIGURE 11
Echocardiogram. The technician is holding a device to the girl's chest. The device sends and receives high-frequency sound waves. It allows the heart to be pictured on the computer screen in front of the technician.

important in reaching a diagnosis. Pneumonia, or other problems of the lungs, is common in infants with heart disease. Chest X-rays are helpful in evaluating these conditions (fig. 10).

A variety of other noninvasive diagnostic studies may be ordered by your cardiologist, depending on the suspected problem. These tests include blood tests, stress tests on a bicycle or treadmill, Holter monitoring (see chapter 6), and echocardiography.

Echocardiography

The echocardiogram has become an extremely useful, noninvasive diagnostic tool. In this test your child lies on an examining table, and electrocardiographic leads are attached.

The room is usually darkened for this test so that the results of the test can be observed on a television screen, which is part of the standard equipment. A technician sits alongside your child and holds an instrument that sounds like an electric razor against your child's chest (fig. 11). This device sends and receives high-frequency sound waves. Echocardiography employs the same technology as sonar, which was developed during World War II to detect submarines and now is used by fishermen to locate schools of fish. It allows a cardiologist to visualize the structure and function of the heart by transmitting and receiving high-frequency ultrasound waves through the heart. It is a painless, extremely useful diagnostic test that is performed essentially without risk.

Echocardiography has reduced the need for invasive testing in certain circumstances, but it is not always a substitute for cardiac catheterization because there is some important information that an echocardiogram cannot provide.

Echocardiography can assist a cardiologist in learning about the size of various heart chambers and the thickness of their walls, about abnormalities in the structure of heart valves and in walls separating the chambers, and about defects in the position and size of the great blood vessels, among other things. The technique has assumed a major role in the diagnosis of heart disease, particularly in infants. In children, echocardiography is also used to assess the function of the heart and to follow the progress of patients after surgery or medical treatment for a heart condition.

Testing During Exercise

Most children are active and like to play, but heart problems may limit the ability to tolerate exercise so that symptoms appear during exertion. In some cases it may be useful to have your child undertake a standard level of exercise under controlled conditions and then measure the response. Only children suspected of having certain kinds of heart problems are usually tested this way.

Your child will exercise using either a treadmill or a bicycle. Either way, continuous exercise is encouraged until fatigue or symptoms appear. During the exercise period, which may last as long as fifteen minutes, the rate of exercise is steadily increased. Your child's heart rate, electrocardiogram, and blood presure are recorded at regular intervals (fig. 12). Your child may also be asked to breathe through a mouthpiece into a specialized device that measures the amount of

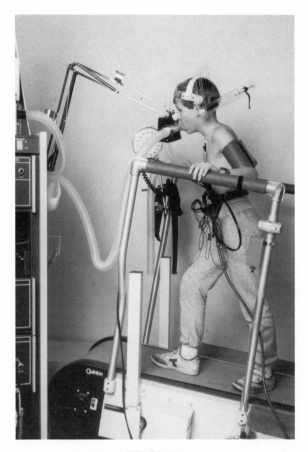

FIGURE 12
Exercise test. The boy is walking on an inclined treadmill. He grips the handrails to stabilize himself. The crownlike device on his head holds the mouthpiece in place.

oxygen he or she is using during exercise and the amount of carbon dioxide being produced. Following exercise, while your child is at rest, measurements continue to be taken until they match the levels recorded before the exercise began. He or she is then asked if anything unusual occurred during the test, for example, pain or dizziness. Your child's participation in this respect is an important element in assessing the results.

In preparing for the exercise session, you should see to it that your child does not eat anything two hours before the test. Light weight clothing and athletic shoes should be worn. Reassure him or her that the degree of exercise will be similar to riding a bicycle vigorously or running a couple of blocks. Your cardiologist will carefully monitor the progress, watching for any adverse effects. The results will be interpreted by comparing your child's response to normal standards for children of the same age and size. The cardiologist can explain what the findings mean. Again, do not be afraid to ask questions.

Reaching a Diagnosis

All information is carefully considered by the cardiologist before a diagnosis is made. Various types of information provide different clues. For example, the patient history may indicate the severity of the disease, whereas murmurs found during the physical examination may suggest that a specific cardiac condition exists. The electrocardiogram and chest X-ray may show the effect of the condition on the heart, and these findings may be confirmed by other measures such as an echocardiogram and an exercise session.

The cardiologist will integrate all this information to reach a diagnosis. The diagnosis may include not only a determination of what heart condition, if any, exists, but also the severity of the condition and, perhaps, what caused it. Once you have been given the diagnosis, the cardiologist will discuss the findings with you in detail. Prepared drawings of the heart problem will sometimes be used to illustrate the location and significance of the defect. You may feel less intimidated and more relaxed talking with a nurse. Once your discussion with the physician has ended, a nurse clinician may be able to meet with you and your child to answer questions and explain further the function of the heart and the particular problem.

It is natural for you to be apprehensive while your child is being evaluated. The goal of a pediatric cardiologist is to arrive at a correct diagnosis and arrange appropriate treatment. Cardiologists try to do this in a nonthreatening manner. In turn, you should try to understand all you can about the problem and what it means so that you can prepare your child—and yourselves—for whatever may need to be done.

The cardiologist virtually never withholds information, even if it is painful or frightening. No purpose would be served by downplaying a serious problem or exaggerating a minor one. Foremost in a cardiologist's mind is the desire to assist you, the parents, in dealing with your child's heart problem effectively. That is why pediatric cardiologists are concerned not only with the medical problem but also with your child as an individual and as a member of your family.

Chapter 3
CARDIAC
CATHETERIZATION

In the next several chapters you will meet Kevin, James, and Erica, young people with heart defects who are being treated successfully. Although each has a unique defect, they have one thing in common: they have undergone cardiac catheterization. This is a procedure in which a tiny, flexible tube called a catheter is introduced into the heart to help the cardiologist make a diagnosis or, occasionally, to help correct a problem. For Kevin, James, and Erica, cardiac catheterization was a key factor in their diagnosis and treatment.

Your cardiologist may recommend this procedure because catheterization is considered the gold standard among diagnostic tests that study the heart and circulation. It provides better and often more detailed information about the structure and function of the heart than any other test. When new, noninvasive tests are developed, their accuracy and utility are invariably compared with the results obtained by cardiac catheterization, which is an invasive procedure.

Not all children with heart disease need cardiac catheterization. But many children who need heart surgery have catheterization performed before the operation. It is not difficult to understand why. During a heart operation, the surgeon cannot waste valuable time searching for a defect. Catheterization can tell the cardiac surgeon what kind of defect exists and exactly where it is. The actual effect of the condition on the heart and the circulatory system can be assessed reliably only by catheterization. Information from the procedure is also useful in determining how well the heart will function after the operation. In short, the success of the operation depends on exact knowledge obtained beforehand. Cardiac catheterization may also be recommended six to twelve months after heart surgery, particularly if the repair was complex, to find out exactly how successful the surgery was and whether further surgery is necessary.

Getting Prepared

Cardiologists occasionally find that parents worry as much about catheterization as they do about an operation. The risk of injury from catheterization is slight and does not justify undue concern. Better understanding of the procedure should alleviate misconceptions about it.

Preparation for catheterization involves you, your child, and the cardiologist responsible for his or her care. Your cardiologist and, at times, your family doctor, will prepare you and your child for the test by explaining its risks and benefits. You need this information to decide whether you want to have it done.

Some typical questions about catheterization are:

> Why is cardiac catheterization being recommended?
> When should it be scheduled?
> How long does it take?
> What are the risks?
> Will my child be hospitalized?
> Is it uncomfortable?
> Will it cause psychological problems?
> Who will perform it?

The cardiologist will discuss these matters with you before making preparations. An educational booklet or videotape about the procedure may be available to answer your questions. We have developed a pamphlet in story form especially for children three to twelve years old. You can learn from such material as well.

The explanation level appropriate for your child obviously depends on his or her age and ability to comprehend. There is no point for a cardiologist to dwell on the potentially uncomfortable aspects of catheterization. But it is not proper to withhold important facts that your child is capable of understanding.

A few days before the scheduled catheterization, tell your child that he or she will be going to the hospital for a special test. Do this in a matter-of-fact way. If you show anxiety, it will be transmitted to your child. You should be honest about what the test involves, but not vivid; detailed descriptions of the procedure are unnecessary and may be harmful. Use booklets and toy doctor kits to help explain it. Do not mislead your child by saying there will be no pain or shots. Be reassuring and say that the test is necessary for him or her to get better and that the doctors and nurses are there to help.

Many cardiac centers admit children to the hospital the day before catheterization is scheduled, although in some settings admission is arranged for early on the day of the procedure. The cardiologist who will perform the catheterization will reexamine your child and talk briefly with you to be certain you have no further questions about what is to be done and why.

You should realize that the cardiologist doing the procedure may not be the same one who examined your child in the clinic and scheduled the catheterization. In many large centers, cardiologists with particular interest and expertise perform all catheterizations.

As we mentioned before, just as you and your child have been counseled regarding the procedure, the physicians involved in the care of your child have likewise prepared. Cardiac catheterization is not like some tests that are always done the same way. Your child's cardiologist discusses his or her case beforehand to determine exactly what information is needed and how that information is best obtained. This is usually done in a conference in which each case scheduled for that week is discussed in detail. The physician who will perform the catheterization makes notes about your child's heart condition and what information must be obtained.

You will be asked to sign a consent form stating that you understand the potential risks and benefits of catheterization. In addition, the cardiologist will often document his or her perception of your understanding in the hospital record.

Your child will not be given anything to eat or drink for a few hours prior to catheterization—the length of time varies depending on his or her age. About forty-five minutes before the procedure is scheduled to begin, a sedative will be administered.

You may be concerned that your infant or child will be frightened and will cry uncontrollably throughout the procedure. As you probably know, children are often better behaved when they are away from their parents. But rest assured that pediatric cardiologists are

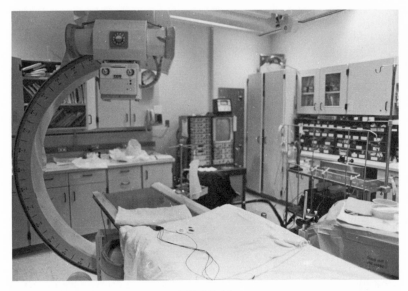

FIGURE 13
Cardiac catheterization laboratory. X-ray equipment is mounted in the C-shaped apparatus, and the table for the patient slides through it. Recording devices and storage areas appear in the background.

experienced in dealing with children of all ages; they know how to calm them and allay their fears.

Catheterization can be done only when the child is in a quiet, resting state, and premedication almost always accomplishes this. When it does not, additional medication is administered in the catheterization laboratory. General anesthesia usually is not used because it adds unnecessarily to the overall risk.

A Wiry Sleuth

Catheterization is usually done in a special room next to the X-ray or surgery departments that has X-ray and other equipment (fig. 13). The procedure is done under sterile conditions. The personnel involved all wear caps, masks, and gowns. Your child will be greeted at the laboratory by a nurse or technician who is ex-

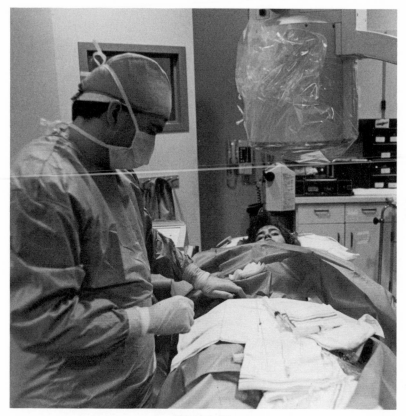

FIGURE 14

Cardiac catheterization. The child undergoing the procedure is positioned on the catheterization table. The cardiologist is preparing to insert the catheter into the groin. The area surrounding the point of insertion has been draped with cloths.

perienced in preparing children for catheterization. This preparation takes about fifteen minutes.

Electrodes are then attached to your child's arms and legs for continuous monitoring of the electrocardiogram. His or her groin is scrubbed with an antiseptic soap, and sterile drapes are applied around the area where the catheter will be inserted. By the time the cardiologist is ready to begin the procedure, your child will probably have fallen asleep from the effects of sedation. The only part of catheterization that is uncomfortable is when the catheter is inserted. The skin surrounding the point of entry is numbed with a local anesthetic, the kind dentists often use (fig. 14). In fact, the level of discomfort is similar to what you experience when a dentist numbs your teeth. This feeling is described to your child as being "like a bee sting."

The cardiologist gains access to the circulatory system by inserting a needle through the numbed skin into the desired blood vessel. Then a guide wire is introduced into the blood vessel and the needle is withdrawn. A thin-walled tube or sheath is advanced over the guide wire into the blood vessel for a distance of several inches. The sheath is designed so that different catheters can easily be inserted or replaced without loss of blood. Once the sheath is in place, there is no further discomfort. Your child will not feel the catheter being manipulated through the blood vessels or heart.

The catheter is advanced through the blood vessel into the heart. The cardiologist watches its course on a fluoroscopic X-ray screen, which is like the screen on a television set. Cardiac catheterization in children usually involves maneuvering the catheter into each of the chambers of the heart and the major arteries and veins that connect to the heart. This is done by gently twisting and probing the catheter while the cardiologist observes it on the television screen. Throughout the procedure a technician monitors the electrocardiogram and tells the cardiologist if changes occur.

Each catheterization procedure differs, depending on the diagnosis and the information needed. Three components are basic: (1) recording pressure in various cardiac chambers and great vessels; (2) analyzing small amounts of blood obtained from these chambers and vessels to determine the oxygen content; and (3) injecting dye through the catheter to visualize a defect, an obstruction, or the size of a chamber. The dye is tracked while it courses through the chambers and major vessels connected to the heart by a special X-ray machine that operates like a movie camera.

The film, which is in black and white, is called a cine angiogram or sometimes cine for short (fig. 15). The dye used for the cine will cause your child to feel a surge of warmth that lasts for several seconds following the injection.

The entire procedure lasts anywhere from thirty minutes to several hours depending on the complexity of the condition and whether special, additional studies are performed. These may in

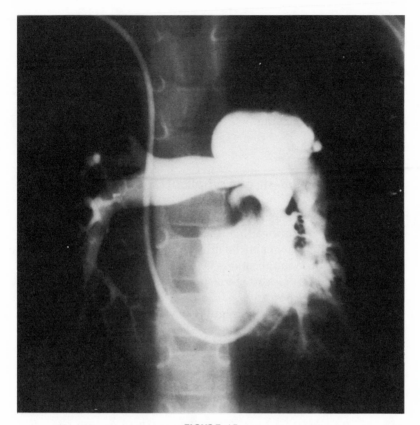

FIGURE 15

Cine Angiogram. Dye, which appears white, has been injected into the right side of the heart. The inside of the right ventricle and pulmonary artery are visible.

clude measuring blood pressures and checking blood samples during exercise, while your child peddles a bicycle attached to the end of the catheterization table, testing the heart as medications are introduced, or studying the electrophysiology of the heart (see chapter 6).

When the study is completed, the catheter is withdrawn through the sheath, and the sheath is removed from the blood vessel. Pressure is applied over the groin for several minutes so that bleeding will not occur, and a pressure bandage is applied. Later in the day, after having reviewed the data and films from the catheterization, the cardiologist will talk to you about the results. At this time, he or she will often let you know if further treatment is required. You may be invited to view the cine angiogram with the cardiologist. Your child will be discharged from the hospital either that evening or the following morning.

Risk of Complications

The risks associated with cardiac catheterization depend on your child's age, his or her health at the time, and, to some degree, the type of defect. In reasonably healthy children more than a year old, the risk of serious complications is less than 0.1 percent, or one in every thousand cardiac catheterizations. The risk for a sick newborn is approximately 2 percent.

Complications include an irregular heartbeat, passage of the catheter through the wall of the heart or a blood vessel, excessive bleeding, induction of a "tetrad spell" (see chapter 4), or infection. Although each of these complications is potentially serious, the staff in the catheterization laboratory is prepared to recognize and deal with them if they occur. Treatment is usually effective.

Some parents do not want to know the risk of the procedure. Their attitude is "if it has to be done, do it and don't talk to me about possible complications." The law and medical ethics require your physician to discuss the risk with you, certainly not to frighten you but to make sure that you are able to give informed consent to the procedure.

In certain cases, cardiac catheterization is used not only to diagnose the condition but also to treat it. For example, if a newborn infant's major heart vessels are transposed or switched, a balloon atrial septostomy is done (see "Transposition of the Great Vessels," chapter 4). With this technique, a hole is created in the atrial septum with a special balloon catheter so that red or saturated blood can get from the left side of the heart to the right side, which pumps blood to the aorta. The procedure is often lifesaving. Certain types of valvular obstruction can also be relieved by inflation of special balloon-tipped catheters. These therapeutic procedures add slightly to the risk of the catheterization but are performed because the risk is less than it would be for an operation.

Chapter 4
CONGENITAL
HEART DISEASE

Kevin is a 28-year-old success story. He is an up-and-coming advertising manager of a large retail company and a member of MENSA, an organization of people with high IQs. Kevin is remarkable because he has succeeded despite a serious congenital heart disease. From kindergarten to the time he graduated from high school, he missed about a third of schooltime. When he was not in school he was at home, protected from extreme temperatures and germs.

"When Kevin was two and a half we took him to a cardiologist," his mother said. "We were told that he had a heart defect and that 90 percent of patients with this particular defect were dead before they were one year old. Nothing could be done. No one asked us, 'Are you all right?' I remember I cried all the way home from the hospital. After a while my husband and I thought that maybe he was born to us because we could give him the special love and care he needed."

Kevin was kept on antibiotics throughout his boyhood so he would not come down with an infection. He was cyanotic now and then, had a poor appetite, and was underweight. He had cardiac catheterization three times. In 1978, when he was twenty, his cardiologist told him that surgery was now an option. Kevin told his counselor that he had decided to "go for broke."

His surgery was a success. "Right now he's real stable," his mother said. "They say things will begin to deteriorate and that someday he will need a heart-lung transplant. That won't be for ten or fifteen years."

"People don't realize how having a child with a heart defect can restructure your life," she said. "I decided I can handle things better when I know what's going on and can share my experiences."

Twelve years ago, when Kevin was sixteen, his mother formed a support *group for parents of children with heart defects, one of a number of such groups around the country (see Appendix D). "I owe a debt for my son," she said.*

Kevin is a survivor of congenital heart disease, an abnormality of the heart that typically develops in the fetus within the first three months of pregnancy. During this period, the heart is assuming its final form. If the heart fails to develop properly at any stage, it will have an abnormal structure that may lead to congenital heart disease.

Congenital heart disease occurs in one of every one hundred infants. About twenty-five thousand babies with congenital heart disease are born in the United States each year, thirty-five hundred in Canada, and seven thousand in the United Kingdom. Although the defect is present at birth, it may not be recognized until days, months, or even years afterward. In many patients the heart disease is mild and requires no treatment. In others an operation is necessary but can be performed with low risk. Among the remaining patients, symptoms develop in early infancy and more extensive treatment or operation is required.

Many parents wonder why their child has a heart problem. In 90 percent of congenital heart defect cases, the cause remains unknown. When we consider how complex the embryonic development of the heart is, it is amazing that more babies are not born with a defect. Yet often when parents learn that their child has such a defect, they blame themselves and think they did something wrong during the pregnancy.

A number of studies have been carried out in an effort to discover factors that might bring about congenital heart disease, but few of these factors have been identified. It has been known for a long time that pregnant women should adopt a sensible diet, maintain good health, and avoid smoking and excessive use of alcohol. Studies have shown that smoking is associated with a lower birth weight and heavy drinking with congenital heart disease.

The Genetic Factor

In most cases, such as Kevin's, congenital heart disease is sporadic, meaning that it does not recur in subsequent children and that there are no instances of other cases in the family. But heredity does appear to play a role in certain families. These families may have more than one child or family member with a congenital defect of the heart. If such a family has one affected child, the chance of having a second is about one in thirty-five.

The incidence of congenital heart disease is likewise higher among the offspring of an affected parent. In families in which more than one member has a heart defect, another affected member is likely to have a defect similar to that in the first family member. Sometimes, when a family learns that a child has congenital heart disease, they begin to volunteer information about heart disease in family members. Half of all Americans die of cardiovascular disease, usually of heart attacks. Keep in mind that congenital heart disease is not the same, and that there is no relationship between heart disease in older people, such as high blood pressure and heart attacks, and congenital heart disease.

Congenital heart disease occurs at a higher frequency in children with other birth defects in which more than one organ is involved, such as Down's syndrome. Congenital heart disease may also be caused by a viral infection in the pregnant woman. However, the only clear-cut relationship that has been shown is between rubella or German measles occurring in the woman during her first three months of pregnancy and congenital cardiac disease.

Classification of the type of congenital heart disease can be difficult. There are at least a hundred forms or variations. Furthermore, it is possible for more than one form to exist in the same child. And each type may produce different symptoms. Another factor confusing the classification is that, in some cases, the abnormality corrects itself as the child grows, and in others the problem changes.

We cannot discuss all these variations in detail, but we shall describe several of the most common malformations of the heart, their features, and the treatment often prescribed. Other defects are described in appendix C.

Your child may have a form of congenital heart disease that is not included in the appendix. We have provided a diagram of the heart (see figure 16) that your physician can use to show you the particular malformation that your child has. Your doctor may also be able to compare the conditions in your child's heart to one of those described in this book.

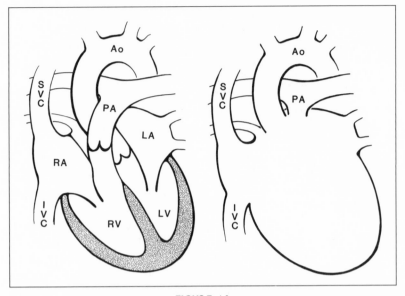

FIGURE 16
Left: Normal heart with major chambers and blood vessels. Right: Heart without valves and walls. (SVC = superior vena cava, IVC = inferior vena cava, RA = right atrium, Ao = aorta, PA = pulmonary artery, RV = right ventricle, LA = left atrium, LV = left ventricle)

Ventricular Septal Defect

In a ventricular septal defect (VSD), there is a hole in the septum or wall separating the pumping chambers, the ventricles (fig. 17). Because the pressure is higher in the left than in the right ventricle, blood flows through the hole from the left to the right ventricle. As a result, some of the oxygen-rich blood in the left ventricle goes through the hole and recirculates through the lungs.

The size of the hole varies considerably, but it is usually very small, smaller than the circumference of a pencil. These small defects produce few or no symptoms because the small size of the hole limits the amount of blood that can flow through it. In about 5 to 10 percent of the cases, however, the defect is large and children typically develop symptoms of heart failure, often at two to three months of age.

In large defects the blood vessels in the lungs react to the trans-

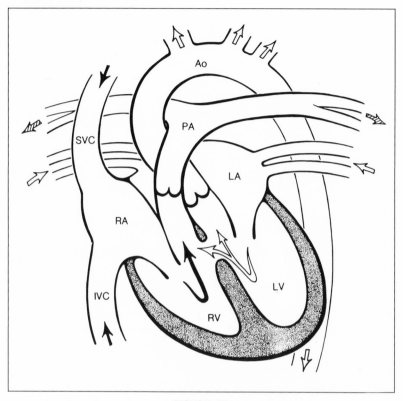

FIGURE 17
Ventricular septal defect. In this anomaly there is a hole in the wall (septum) separating the left ventricle (LV) from the right ventricle (RV). The oxygen-poor blood (dark arrows) flows normally through the superior vena cava (SVC) and inferior vena cava (IVC) into the right atrium (RA), the RV, and the pulmonary artery (PA). The oxygen-rich blood returns to the left atrium (LA) and flows into the LV. Some of the blood from the LV flows normally into the aorta (Ao), but a portion flows through the defect and recirculates through the lungs.

mission of the high pressure from the left ventricle through the defect into the right side of the heart. This reaction involves a narrowing of the lumen or opening of the small pulmonary arteries in the lungs. This narrowing may initially result from constriction of the blood vessel, but, later, irreversible changes and scarring occur in these arteries. They begin to deteriorate and may narrow to the

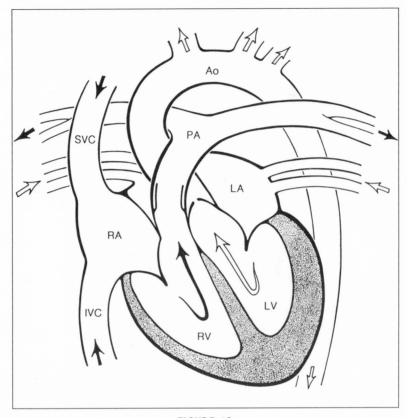

FIGURE 18

Aortic stenosis. Blood flows normally through the right side of the heart
and through the lungs. However, the aortic valve, which separates the left
ventricle (LV) from the aorta (Ao), does not open properly, so the pressure
in the LV rises.

point that the pressure on the right side of the heart exceeds that
on the left side, with the result that blood begins to flow from the
right to the left ventricle. The patient begins to turn blue because
a portion of the unoxygenated blood reaches the aorta. Changes in
the lung shorten the child's life span and increase the risks associated with surgery. Early operations for VSD are designed to
prevent such risks.

A ventricular septal defect is usually found by the presence of a loud murmur at two weeks to two months of age. If this defect is discovered in your child, the cardiologist's recommendation for managing the problem may depend on X-ray and EKG findings and your infant's condition. Those defects that are small require no treatment and the hole will close by itself. Those that are large and produce clear symptoms may be closed surgically or, in the case of multiple defects that may be difficult to reach, by placing a constriction or band on the pulmonary artery. This procedure protects the lungs, improves the condition, and allows your child to grow until he or she is better prepared for surgery. Then the band is removed and the defect closed. Over the years the risk associated with an operative correction has diminished. Improved results make the long-term outlook for children with this defect excellent.

Aortic Stenosis

Aortic stenosis means there is a constriction where blood flows from the left ventricle into the aorta, the large artery that carries blood to be distributed throughout the body (fig. 18). The constriction usually occurs at the aortic valve and is called valvular aortic stenosis. Once in a while there is an obstruction above the aortic valve, supravalvular stenosis, or below the aortic valve, subaortic stenosis.

Regardless of the location of the constriction, it impedes the flow of blood from the left ventricle. To overcome the obstruction, the pressure in the left ventricle increases because the ventricle must pump harder to get blood through this narrow opening. To develop the higher level of pressure needed, the wall of the left ventricle grows thicker or hypertrophies. Some infants have heart failure, and older children may have chest pain, dizziness, or fainting spells. These symptoms indicate severe obstruction. Most infants and children, however, have no symptoms.

Cardiac catheterization has become an important advance in the management of aortic stenosis because with it the pressure in the left ventricle can be measured and abnormally high pressure recorded. Newer echocardiographic techniques also provide important information. Most infants or children with aortic stenosis will ultimately require an operation. In infants with heart failure or chil-

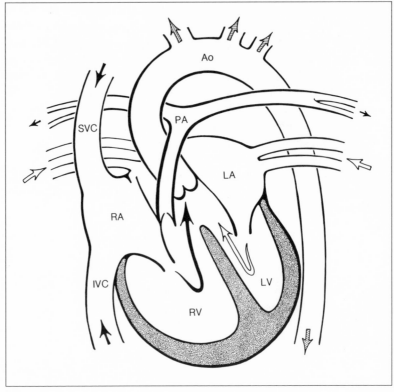

FIGURE 19

Tetralogy of Fallot. In this anomaly there are two major problems. The first is a hole in the wall separating the right ventricle (RV) from the left ventricle (LV). The second is a narrowing in the blood vessel that goes to the pulmonary artery (PA) and on to the lungs. Because of this narrowing, some oxygen-poor blood flows from the RV, through the defect, and into the aorta (Ao).

dren with serious chest pain, surgery should be done as soon as the symptoms occur.

For adolescents who do not have symptoms, cardiologists also recommend widening the opening between the left ventricle and the aorta. Even with treatment and surgery, however, careful, long-term follow-up is necessary because complete relief of the obstruction is unusual. Moreover, the narrowing tends to recur over decades so that a second operation may be required. For some children, participation in rigorous athletic activity or exercise may have to be restricted. If your child has aortic stenosis, you should take measures to prevent heart infection (see "bacterial endocarditis," chapter 5) because he or she is probably at greater risk than are children with other heart anomalies.

Tetralogy of Fallot

Although the prefix tetra suggests four parts, this condition, described by the French physician Fallot, is usually made up of two major defects: a ventricular septal defect, and pulmonary stenosis or an obstruction that interferes with blood flowing into the lungs (fig. 19). Most of the time this obstruction is a severe one: venous (blue) blood passes from the right ventricle directly into the left ventricle and then into the aorta, causing the child to take on a bluish cast characteristic of cyanosis. The other two components of tetralogy of Fallot are a thicker wall in the right ventricle, owing to elevated pressure, and a straddling effect of the aorta at the ventricular septal defect, which makes the aorta appear to arise from both ventricles.

Many children with tetralogy of Fallot become cyanotic during the first year of life. If your child has this condition, he or she may at times begin breathing rapidly and even lose consciousness. These episodes are often frightening and can in fact be life-threatening. During such an episode, you should comfort your child and place him or her in a knee-chest position.

Most children with tetralogy of Fallot require surgery, often one of two types: a surgical shunt is performed (figs. 20 and 21), creating a passage for blood through the typically small pulmonary arteries; or the ventricular septal defect is closed and the obstruction to the lungs relieved, often with a patch. Newer surgical techniques and postoperative management have lowered the risk for these children, and most of them can lead a normal or near-normal life with periodic follow-up examinations to monitor defects, such as residual heart murmur or cardiac enlargement, which may still exist.

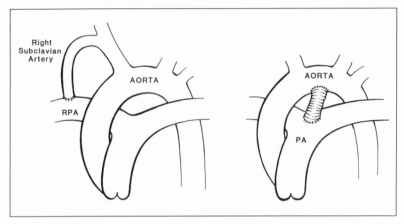

FIGURE 20

Two types of temporizing operations for tetralogy of Fallot and similar conditions. These operations are called shunt operations because they shunt (carry) some blood, which should be going to the body, into the lungs. **Left: Blalock-Taussig.** In this procedure the right subclavian artery, which carries blood to the right arm, is divided and sewn into the right pulmonary artery (RPA). **Right: Central shunt.** In this operation a tube of synthetic material is sewn between the aorta and the pulmonary artery (PA). In both instances blood flows from the high pressure aorta into the lower pressure pulmonary artery.

Transposition of the Great Vessels

Of the infants born with a heart defect, one in every ten suffers from a malformation called transposition of the great vessels (TGV). In this anomaly, the aorta arises from the right ventricle, and the pulmonary artery from the left ventricle — the exact opposite of normal circulation (fig. 22). As a result, two independent circulatory systems exist: in one system blood circulates between the heart and the lungs, and in the other it circulates from the heart through the rest of the body but fails to get oxygen from the lungs. Complete TGV is thus fatal unless another defect allows some mixing of the blood in the two systems.

Newborns with TGV are severely cyanotic and symptoms develop within the first twenty-four hours after birth. Usually no heart murmur is found and the electrocardiogram is indistinguishable

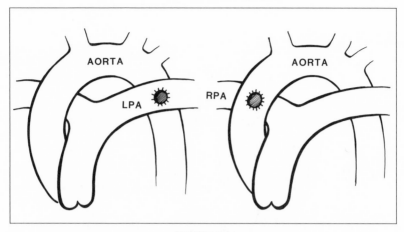

FIGURE 21
Two more temporizing shunt procedures. **Left: Pott's.** In this operation a connection is made between the aorta and the left pulmonary artery (LPA). **Right: Waterston.** In this procedure a connection is made between the aorta and the right pulmonary artery (RPA). In both instances blood flows from the high pressure aorta into the lower pressure pulmonary artery.

from that of a normal infant. Chest X-ray and echocardiography help the cardiologist arrive at a correct diagnosis.

One third of the children with TGV have a ventricular septal defect that permits some oxygenated blood to circulate through the body. In the other two thirds of children with TGV, there is communication between the two circulation systems through the ductus arteriosus, a blood vessel that connects the pulmonary artery to the aorta prior to birth. The ductus usually closes within forty-eight hours of birth. Sometimes a drug can be administered to newborns that helps to keep the ductus arteriosus open and makes possible a procedure to alleviate the critical problem (See "Important Advances in Research," chapter 10). Doctors must create or maintain an opening between the two circulatory sytems.

In this procedure, called balloon atrial septostomy or Rashkind procedure (fig. 23), a balloon-tipped catheter is inserted into the left atrium, inflated, and then forcefully withdrawn across the atrial septum that separates the two sides of the circulatory system. The action tears the atrial septum and permits blood from the two sys-

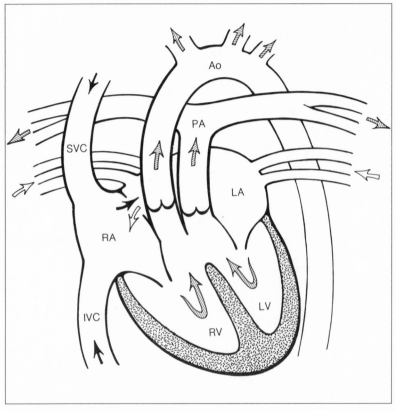

FIGURE 22

Transposition of the great vessels (TGV). In this anomaly the major blood vessels leaving the heart originate from the opposite ventricles than normal. Therefore the aorta (Ao) originates from the right ventricle (RV), and the pulmonary artery (PA) arises from the left ventricle (LV). Thus the oxygen-poor (blue) blood, traveling to the heart through the superior vena cava (SVC) and inferior vena cava (IVC), is returned to the body. Oxygen-rich (red) blood is returned to the left atrium (LA) and is pumped by the LV into the lungs again.

tems to mix. This is a temporizing procedure that maintains adequate circulation and heart function until the child is about a year old, when surgery can be done to establish a normal circulatory pat-

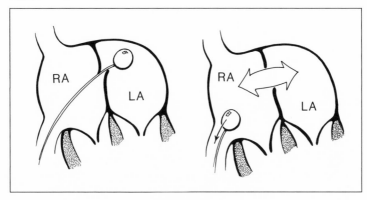

FIGURE 23

Balloon atrial septostomy. (Also called Rashkind procedure.) This procedure is principally used for children with transposition of the great vessels. A catheter is advanced through the inferior vena cava into the left atrium (LA). A balloon on the catheter is inflated and rapidly pulled back into the right atrium (RA). When the catheter is pulled back, it creates an opening in the wall between the atria.

tern. The preferred technique involves creating a baffle or tunnel in the atrium to reverse the circulation at that location. Children with a ventricular septal defect or other abnormality may have to undergo a more complicated procedure that involves the use of a conduit or tube to rechannel blood flow.

Complications may arise following surgery or in the long term: for example, the baffle may scar and constrict the veins; the electrical system in the atria may be injured, causing irregular heartbeat, or the right ventricle may not be capable of developing an adequate pressure to pump blood for a long period, a task normally done by the more powerful left ventricle. These problems are addressed on a case-by-case basis.

The application of new diagnostic, surgical, and treatment techniques has had a greater effect on the outlook of children with TGV than perhaps on those with any other cardiac defect. With continued long-term follow-up, the outlook for patients with this once lethal condition is very good.

Promising Vistas

If your child has a congenital heart defect, he or she will need routine checkups and care by your family physician or pediatrician. Your child may have problems developing normally and more frequent visits may be necessary. In general, regular feeding instructions and diets are recommended by your doctor.

If your child is born with a heart defect, he or she is not unusually susceptible to other illnesses. Special precautions, such as avoiding day care programs and flu vaccine or other types of immunization, are not necessary. Some children with particular types of defects may be prone to pneumonia, particularly during the first year of life. Your child should be treated with antibiotics if the pneumonia is due to bacteria but does not need antibiotics for every cough or cold. Antibiotics should be administered prior to dental or oral surgical procedures, however.

Remarkable strides have been made over the past twenty-five years in the diagnosis and treatment of congenital heart disease. And today there are nearly half a million people in the United States who are able to live with the disease. Often an operation can be done that will correct the condition and permit normal activities. Some cases do not require any treatment. In our long-term studies of affected children, we have found that most of them grow up to lead normal, healthy lives.

We believe that most children with congenital heart disease, even after surgery, require periodic check-ups, perhaps only at five-year intervals. These can help to determine whether any long-term problems may develop and to prepare parents and children for dealing with them if they do.

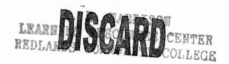
Chapter 5
ACQUIRED HEART DISEASE

James is a typical fifteen-year-old boy in almost every way. He is bright, likable, and often forgetful when it comes to taking his medication. James has a heart defect that developed after he was born. At first his outlook was bleak without surgery. His cardiologist consulted with colleagues about James's unusual problem and decided to put him on a new drug. His condition improved dramatically. Today, ten years later, James is among the most physically fit boys in his class and shows no visible signs of a heart problem. His doctor no longer thinks surgery will be necessary, as long as the medication keeps working.

"Our GP picked up a murmur when James was three-and-a-half years old," his mother said. "He suggested that we wait a year and test him again. We did, and the murmur was still there. So we took him to a cardiologist."

"He was thoroughly evaluated and diagnosed with the same condition I have, subaortic stenosis, only his is more severe," she said. "When James was ten, he was catheterized. The information confirmed that the heart wall had been damaged. We were told of the possibility of valve transplants, which would be put off until he was in his late teens. He was put on propanolol after the catheterization, but he didn't improve. He became depressed. Then his cardiologist put him on another drug. Now the biggest problem is reminding him to take it."

Heart disease may develop after a child is born rather than during fetal development (congenital heart disease). The acquired diseases that attack the heart may affect one or all of its structures: the valves, the endocardium or lining of the heart chambers, the my-

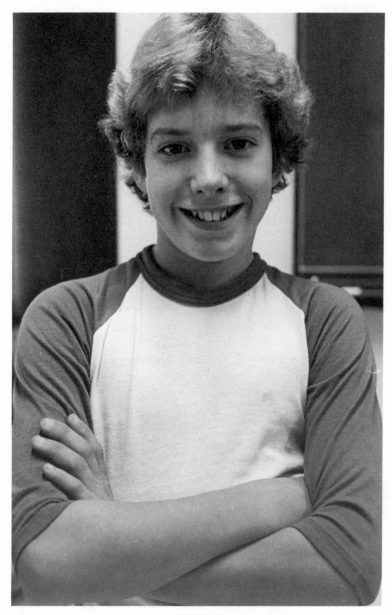

FIGURE 24

James at age fifteen.

ocardium or heart muscle, and the pericardium, the sac around the heart.

Acquired heart diseases may be caused by bacteria or viruses. In some children with an acquired heart disease, such as James, a cause cannot be found. These conditions are called idiopathic and treatment can be difficult. If a specific cause can be determined, the child can usually be treated more successfully.

Many conditions can affect the heart. If your doctor suspects that your child has an acquired heart disease, certain diagnostic tests will be done. They usually include electrocardiogram, chest X-ray, and echocardiogram. A variety of other tests may be ordered, but cardiac catheterization is not as widely used for children with acquired heart disease as it is for those with congenital heart disorders. Doctors can also use different types of blood cultures and muscle biopsy to help determine the cause. When particular problems are encountered, a muscle biopsy is performed in which a tiny piece of the myocardium is removed by catheterization or surgery and analyzed.

Because so many different conditions can affect the heart, only the most common types of acquired heart disease, especially those with a well-defined set of signs and symptoms, are discussed in detail in this chapter. If information specific to your child's condition is not included, your doctor should be able to indicate which portions of this book are appropriate for you or refer you to other sources.

Cardiomyopathy

Cardiomyopathy is a term that refers to a broad range of conditions that affect the heart muscle, the myocardium. The cause of some of these conditions is known, but in most patients, like James, whom we met at the beginning of this chapter, the cause cannot be identified. Faulty metabolism of the heart muscle is one apparent cause, but this tends to be uncommon. In some instances more than one member of a family has cardiomyopathy, so if one of your children is affected, your doctor may want to examine you and your other children. For example, James's mother is affected, but neither of his two brothers have the disease.

The structure of heart muscle resembles the muscle in our arms and legs in many ways. Therefore, it is not surprising that disease affecting muscle in general may also affect the heart muscle. Cardiomyopathy produces similar symptoms and problems in children. The three main problems involving heart muscle are failure of heart function, structure, and electrical system.

A heart with weakened muscle cannot deliver the normal quantity of blood through the body. If your child is affected, he or she tires easily and cannot keep up with other children in active play. As the disease gets worse, your child may be tired constantly. The amount of blood the heart pumps may be so small that he or she has chest pain, fainting spells, and may appear pale and cold with mottled skin. These symptoms are usually accompanied by low blood pressure.

As the heart muscle grows weaker, the heart chambers become dilated, resulting in an enlarged heart. Your doctor can see this enlargement on a chest X-ray. Indeed, one of the ways cardiomyopathy is recognized is discovery of an enlarged heart in a child who has had a chest X-ray for another condition. In a dilated heart, the cardiac valves may leak. Such leakage could result in a murmur. Some children with cardiomyopathy develop arrhythmias, malfunctions of the heart's electrical system, which controls the regular and orderly contraction of the heart chambers (see "Cardiac Arrhythmias," chapter 6). These arrhythmias may be premature beats, tachycardia, or heart block. Cardiac arrythmia is sometimes the initial clue in diagnosing the underlying disease.

Cardiomyopathy has been divided into three groups based on the symptoms and heart structures that are affected. The most common form is congestive cardiomyopathy in which the heart is greatly dilated or enlarged and the child has features of congestive heart failure. Blood flow is restricted and the lungs and abdomen become congested. An enlarged liver is another sign of cardiomegaly.

In obstructive cardiomyopathy, the walls of the heart are dramatically thickened. As a result, the outflow area of the organ is narrowed and obstructed. The pressure in the ventricles may be twice what is normal. Affected children usually have an adequate output of blood flow but may suffer episodes of chest pain or fainting.

In restrictive cardiomyopathy, a third form of the disease, the chamber walls are thickened and smaller than normal. This limits the amount of blood that can flow into the ventricles, producing symptoms similar to those just described.

Cardiomyopathy is most easily diagnosed by echocardiography.

This is a sensitive method for detecting the overall condition of the heart and the particular type of cardiomyopathy. In some cases, cardiac catheterization can furnish additional, useful information. A special catheter can be advanced into the heart to obtain a minute piece of heart muscle that can be analyzed in an attempt to find a cause.

At present, there is no treatment or cure for cardiomyopathy itself. Only the symptoms are treated. For example, if a child has congestive heart failure as a result of the disease, digitalis and a diuretic are administered. Digitalis is a powerful cardiac stimulant widely prescribed for adults with a history of heart problems. Diuretics help the body eliminate retained fluid that poses a burden for the heart. Medicine may be given to reduce an obstruction if one is present, but the results are variable. At some medical centers, surgery is performed to help relieve such obstructions in children having characteristic symptoms.

Rheumatic Fever

You have probably heard of rheumatic fever, and certainly your parents have. In their youth, rheumatic fever was very common in the United States, much like tuberculosis.

Until recently, about one in two hundred thousand white children got rheumatic fever every year. This is an extremely low figure. Today clusters of cases have been found in population groups in several areas of the United States. The rate is higher in impoverished children who are less likely to receive the medical care and education needed to prevent the disease.

Rheumatic fever is an acute disease caused by a strep throat infection. Strep is the shortened name for the bacteria streptococcus. This bacteria can infect the tonsils, causing tonsillitis, and the throat, causing a sore throat or pharyngitis. With strep throat, there is fever, usually about 101 degrees Fahrenheit or greater, and the lymph glands in the neck are swollen and tender. The affected child may have a headache and appear ill. During a lifetime, a person may get as many as twenty-five strep infections, but only in a rare instance will one of them cause rheumatic fever.

Rheumatic fever typically begins a week or two after a strep infection. After the child has apparently recovered from the symptoms of strep and returned to school, he or she suddenly comes down with a fever again but without a sore throat accompanying it. Fatigue, lack of appetite, and sore joints are other symptoms.

Rheumatic fever may affect the heart along with other organs. Not all children who get the disease will have heart problems, but these problems are very serious because they may result in permanent and progressive changes that can lead to complications requiring treatment.

Any part of the heart may be involved. For example, inflammation of the heart valves can eventually cause them to "leak," and later, when scarring occurs, to become constricted. Damaged valves can lead to heart murmurs. A doctor must distinguish such murmurs from those normal murmurs described in chapter 2. A characteristic murmur is the most common diagnostic feature of rheumatic heart disease.

Less often, the heart muscle (myocardium) or sac around the heart (pericardium) may be affected. Special tests may be needed, such as electrocardiogram or chest X-ray, to diagnose these disorders. If the myocardium is involved, the heart shadow appears enlarged on the X-ray. If the disease is severe, the X-ray may indicate congestive heart failure. Pericarditis, or inflammation of the pericardium, may cause sharp chest pain and show up on the electrocardiogram. In most children with rheumatic fever, myocarditis and pericarditis resolve themselves and do not produce permanent changes. In a few, however, they can have severe and occasionally fatal consequences.

Rheumatic fever can lead to acute arthritis in the large joints: the hips, knees, ankles, shoulders, elbows, or wrists. The condition is called migratory arthritis because first one and then another joint is affected. An affected joint is red, swollen, and tender. Movement is painful. For example, a child whose knee joints are inflamed will avoid walking. The symptoms will disappear very rapidly with aspirin, usually within twenty-four hours, and the affected joints will not be permanently damaged.

In a few cases, particularly in adolescents, the brain is affected by rheumatic fever. The resulting symptoms can be disconcerting and have been called chorea or St. Vitus's Dance. Affected children become emotionally upset and may cry easily. They develop purposeless, random motions that range from fidgety behavior to sudden dramatic movements. School performance lags and handwriting deteriorates during the acute episode. These symptoms will pass after a few months and children usually recover with no permanent disabilities.

Once in a while, rheumatic fever affects the skin. One manifestation is called erythema marginatum. This is a red rash, usually somewhere on the trunk of the body. The rash is clearly outlined and will gradually expand and then disappear, sometimes all within twenty minutes. Heat, as from a hot bath, may bring out the rash.

Diagnosis of rheumatic fever rests upon a well-defined set of signs and symptoms called the Jones Criteria. These criteria were developed by the American Heart Association to assist physicians in reaching a diagnosis and to avoid misdiagnosis or overdiagnosis. They are based on information gathered from an examination and from various laboratory tests.

The first requirement for the diagnosis is evidence of a streptococcal infection, indicated by the presence of strep on a throat culture or, better yet, by signs that the body has reacted to strep by forming antibodies against it. The other features include evidence that specific organs, such as the heart, brain, or skin, have been affected, or that a generalized condition of inflammation exists. This condition can be detected by a blood test. If your child is diagnosed as having rheumatic fever, he or she will probably be hospitalized until inflammation subsides, and then your child will be allowed to increase activity gradually. Several months may pass before a full level of activity can be resumed.

To combat inflammation, aspirin is administered in rather large doses. Blood is drawn regularly to help keep medication at the optimal level. In severe cases, cortisone is given. As the signs of inflammation decrease, the medication is gradually reduced and then withdrawn. In an acute episode, your child will be treated with penicillin for the streptococcal infection. While in the hospital, periodic blood tests, electrocardiograms, and chest X-rays may be undertaken to evaluate the disease process.

After your child is discharged from the hospital, periodic examinations and blood tests will be required as he or she begins to resume normal activity. This may occur over a period of three months. If the heart was affected during the acute episode, scarring of the heart valves may occur over a period of decades. The scarred valves may narrow, obstructing the blood flow, or they may be held open so that they leak. In these circumstances, further treatment, and possibly surgery, is necessary.

Once your child has had an episode of acute rheumatic fever, he or she is more likely to have a second episode. Patients who have such episodes have to take penicillin regularly for the rest of their lives. The penicillin is administered either in the form of tablets daily or by injection monthly. Continuous penicillin prevents streptococcal infections and the recurrence of rheumatic fever.

Most cases of sore throat and tonsillitis are not due to strep, and in fact most sore throats do not require treatment with penicillin or antibiotics. Your doctor may perform a throat culture on your child to determine if strep is present. To do this, the throat is swabbed and the substance obtained is plated on a special growth material. Identification of the bacterium takes twenty-four hours. If your doctor suspects the presence of strep, he or she will prescribe penicillin at the same time the culture is obtained. If the culture does not show strep, the medication is discontinued.

Bacterial Endocarditis

Bacterial endocarditis is an infection of the lining of the heart, the endocardium. It is an uncommon but serious complication of other forms of heart disease, such as valvular or congenital heart disease.

Bacteria pass into our blood stream at different times and in different ways, often via a cut, wound, or incision. They may enter when the dentist works on our teeth. Bacteria normally present in our mouths can enter the bloodstream, just as they may during a tonsillectomy or treatment of an infected toenail. They pass through the heart and are quickly eliminated by the body's defense mechanisms.

If your child has an abnormal heart valve or an opening between the heart chambers, such as a ventricular septal defect, the bacteria can become lodged in the abnormal tissue. There they grow and multiply, establishing an infection within the heart. A heart infection is serious because it can erode the organ's major vessels. In some cases small pieces of infected material called emboli break off and pass to other organs where they cause other complications.

Bacterial endocarditis is suspected when your child is known to have a heart defect and has had persistent fever for no apparent reason. A fever in a child with a normal heart will last a couple days at most, regardless of the cause. With bacterial endocarditis, the fever lasts for several days and your child may run a temperature of up to 103 degrees Fahrenheit. The fever is sometimes accompanied by chills, weariness, and lack of appetite.

In examining your child, the cardiologist will listen for a murmur, a change reflecting erosion of heart tissue from infection. In addition, evidence of emboli that have passed to other sites will be searched for, under the fingernails, for example, where small hemorrhages that resemble splinters may be noticed, or in the abdomen, where an enlarged spleen may mean that the infected material has spread there.

Laboratory work can help in making a diagnosis. The hemoglobin value may be low. When there is infection or inflammation, protein in the blood causes a sample that has been allowed to sit to settle faster. There may be red blood cells in a urine sample, indicating that emboli have passed to the kidneys.

The key to diagnosis of bacterial endocarditis is in blood cultures. Several samples of blood are drawn and attempts made to grow the bacteria from the blood. If bacterial growth is successful and analysis of symptoms is complete, the diagnosis can be confirmed. The type of bacterium can be identified and its susceptibility to antibiotics determined.

Treatment of bacterial endocarditis requires a prolonged hospitalization of one to two months. Most infections take at least six weeks to treat. Following the course, your child may be kept in the hospital a few days to make certain the infection has subsided.

Large doses of antibiotics are used to combat the infection. In many cases they are injected at first and later administered orally. The types of antibiotics are selected very carefully, depending on the type of bacteria and their susceptibility to the antibiotic. During treatment, your child will be evaluated repeatedly to detect possible destructive effects on the heart or the effects of emboli on various organs.

Bacterial endocarditis is a very serious infection. Up to 10 percent of patients die. If a valve is so eroded that it leaks excessively, an operation may be required to replace it. There may be complications produced by emboli. However, most patients survive without developing complications. Your child is most susceptible if he or she has a known heart condition, but measures can be taken to help prevent this insidious infection (see p. 62).

Kawasaki Disease

Kawasaki disease is an acute inflammation perhaps caused by an infectious agent, possibly a virus, and named after the Japanese pediatrician who first described it in 1967. Kawasaki disease is most common in Japan, but during the past decade cases have been reported in the United States and other countries. The disease typically affects children between three and four years old.

One of the complications of Kawasaki disease is damage to the arteries from inflammation. Inflammation weakens the walls of the arteries, causing them to form tiny bulges called aneurysms. Arteries in the arms or abdomen may be affected. If the coronary arteries are involved, the disease can be fatal. It is possible for these aneurysms to rupture, leading to hemorrhage. If the coronary arteries become clotted, the heart muscle can be damaged, as in a heart attack. Although only about 2 percent of children with Kawasaki disease develop this complication of the coronary arteries, those showing symptoms should be evaluated by a cardiologist.

The major features of the disease are: fever lasting as long as three weeks, with wide, daily swings; inflamed eyes and eyelids, reddish tongue, lips, and throat; swollen hands and feet with reddened palms and soles and subsequent peeling, particularly on the fingertips; a red rash on the trunk of the body; and enlarged lymph nodes in the neck.

There is little difficulty in diagnosing Kawasaki disease when these features are present, but you may become alarmed if your child develops a fever without an apparent cause. The doctor can run several tests to identify a cause. Actually, there are no diagnostic blood tests for Kawasaki disease. It is typical, however, for the white blood count and platelet count to be elevated severalfold as a response to inflammation.

The cardiologist will initially perform an electrocardiogram and a chest X-ray. The electrocardiogram may show changes in the heart muscle and the chest X-ray cardiac enlargement. An echocardiogram will show dilation of the coronary arteries.

Most aneurysms of the coronary arteries occur near their origin from the aorta. This is the part of the coronary arteries that is best seen on an echocardiogram. Echocardiography is a fairly sensitive method of detecting aneurysms. At some medical centers, cardiac catheterization is done. The catheter is passed into the aorta, and an angiogram is undertaken to demonstrate the size and appearance of the coronary arteries.

There is no specific drug or antibiotic to treat Kawasaki disease. It is generally treated with aspirin. Even with the high doses used to combat inflammation, response to treatment is slow. This is often frustrating, for it may take a couple of weeks for the fever to subside.

After the acute phase of the illness, the aspirin dose is reduced to low levels, thereby reducing the chances of blood clots forming in the coronary arteries. Another medication, Persantin, may be used for the same purpose. Prolonged use of aspirin is not needed if the coronary arteries are not affected. With prolonged therapy the coronary arteries may return to normal.

Several recent studies indicate that Kawasaki disease may be caused by a special type of virus called a retrovirus. If these studies are confirmed, they could lead to better diagnosis and possibly a vaccine.

Mitral Valve Prolapse

Mitral valve prolapse has also been called floppy mitral valve or Barlow syndrome, after the cardiologist who first called attention to it. You recall from chapter 1 that there are four heart valves. One of these, called the mitral valve, separates the left atrium and left ventricle.

If your child has mitral valve prolapse, when the leaflets of the mitral valve close, they protrude or prolapse back into the left atrium. If they seal shut, there is no problem. Once in a while, however, the valve protrudes to such an extent that the leaflets no longer shut tight, allowing blood to leak from the left ventricle into the left atrium. This is called mitral valve insufficiency or mitral regurgitation.

In recent years, mitral valve prolapse is being diagnosed more frequently, particularly with the development of echocardiography. When echocardiographic surveys are done, up to 7 percent of adolescents or young adults show some signs of this mitral valve anomaly. Most of them have no symptoms and their condition cannot be detected by routine examination. In fact, most people who have a mild case of mitral valve prolapse will never know they have it and will suffer no consequences. Even with a murmur, the outlook is excellent, and the condition does not worsen. Vague chest pain or episodes of irregular heartbeat may be the only noticeable effects.

Children who show mitral valve prolapse on an echocardiogram do not need treatment. Furthermore, we believe these children are better off if they do not know about it. For children with a murmur, the only requirement is to prevent bacterial endocarditis, which can be done with antibiotics. They do not need to be restrained from physical activity. In the occasional child with chest pain or irregular heartbeat, a medication called propranolol is usually prescribed. Propranolol belongs to a class of drugs called beta blockers that slow the heart rate and weaken the force of ventricular contraction.

Pericarditis

Pericarditis is an inflammation of the sac around the heart, the pericardium. It may be caused by an infection, usually a virus, but occasionally in infants by a bacterium. Bacterial pericarditis is a very serious problem. Diseases that cause generalized inflammation, such as rheumatic fever or rheumatoid arthritis, may be associated with it. Benign heart tumors and kidney failure have also been linked to pericarditis. Most children develop the condition following open heart surgery because the pericardial sac is opened during the operation. In some cases, however, the cause of pericarditis is never found.

Pericarditis may be painful. Indeed, the chest pain caused by inflammation of the pericardium is the most common and obvious symptom. A second problem is that the inflamed pericardium may leak fluid into the pericardial sac, a situation doctors refer to as pericardial effusion. If a large amount of fluid collects, it can compress the heart and seriously impair its function.

Yet another problem occurs in those infants with bacteria in the pericardial sac. They may become very ill and even die. Once in a while the heart sac may scar over a period of years following an acute episode. Such scarring can compress the heart, resulting in a chronic illness called constrictive pericarditis or cardiac tamponade, a condition in which the neck veins are often distended and the heartbeat sounds muffled.

If your infant has bacterial pericarditis, he or she probably has a high-grade fever and appears very sick. The cardiologists making a diagnosis will pay particular attention to the blood pressure and pulse rate, for when pericardial tamponade is developing, blood pressure can drop to dangerously low levels and the pulse rate is abnormally high.

When listening to your infant's heart, your doctor may hear a characteristic grating noise called a pericardial rub. This occurs when the inflamed pericardia rub together. Echocardiography may be done to detect pericardial effusion because it can easily detect a buildup of fluid around the heart. If pericardial effusion is serious, a pericardial tap is performed. Under sterile conditions, a needle is placed beneath the breastbone into the pericardial sac and the fluid is drained. This fluid is carefully analyzed to determine the cause of the inflammation.

Many children do not require treatment, and in some instances specific treatment is not available. Usually pericarditis improves as the basic condition causing the inflammation improves. Children with fever are given aspirin or cortisone. If the infection is found to be caused by a bacterium, large doses of antibiotics are administered. In cases in which a tamponade has developed, a tube is inserted and the fluid is drained.

Chapter 6
CARDIAC
ARRHYTHMIAS

The heart comes as close to perfection as any pump imaginable. Think of it: five thousand beats per hour, more than one hundred thousand beats per day, and more than two billon beats in an average lifetime. But nature is not perfect; some children have irregular heartbeats.

During an examination your doctor may find that your child's heartbeat is irregular. Perhaps your child already told you about a funny "flip-flop" feeling in his or her chest. Such irregularities of the heartbeat are called arrhythmias. Because the living heart is never without some form of rhythm, another term for conditions of abnormal rhythm is dysrhythmia. These two terms, arrhythmia and dysrhythmia, are often used interchangeably.

As described in chapter 1, the orderly contraction of the heart is controlled by unique cells that make up specialized conduction tissue, resembling an electrical circuit. The speed and regularity of the heartbeat are regulated by the sinoatrial or sinus (SA) node, the small nodule of tissue in the roof of the right atrium. The SA node, in turn, is regulated by chemical messengers released by certain glands after a command from the brain.

An electrical impulse is generated by the SA node when it fires, spreading through the pathways in the atria and causing them to contract. These impulses converge in a second small nodule, the atrioventricular (AV) node, located where the atria join the ventricles. The impulse slowly passes through the AV node, allowing time for the atrium to contract to fill the ventricles with blood. The impulse then spreads down the bundle of His into the ventricles, causing them to contract simultaneously and completing the orderly sequence of the heartbeat.

Most children with an abnormal heart rate or rhythm have an otherwise normal heart. Irregular heartbeat in children is sometimes caused by congenital abnormalities of the conduction tissue rather than by an acquired disease. Other causes include viruses that infect the heart, abnormal levels of sodium or potassium in the blood, and diseases of heart muscle.

Now and then a child is born with immature and incompletely formed SA or AV tissue. This is the most common cause of irregular heartbeat in the first three months of life. Such irregularities are often passing and tend to disappear when the conduction system matures. They may require treatment initially, but they do not recur later in childhood.

The most common cause of an abnormal heartbeat in children is a condition called accessory conduction pathway (fig. 25). The atria and ventricles are normally connected by a single pathway, that of the AV node. If another pathway connecting the atria and ventricles besides the AV node exists, an impulse can take that pathway. The additional pathway allows an impulse that has passed normally from the atrium to the ventricle through the AV node to take the accessory pathway from the ventricles back into the atrium. This excites the atrium and the impulse then reenters the ventricle, creating a circular conduction mechanism. Children with this problem have a heart that beats very rapidly, perhaps three hundred times a minute or four to five times the normal rate. Less commonly, the impulse travels in the opposite direction—downward from the atria through the accessory conduction tissue and back up through the AV node, with the same results.

Another cause of arrhythmia is maldevelopment of or injury to the SA node. Usually this problem is not a dangerous one. When the connection between the AV node and the bundle of His is absent, however, the heart rate is seriously slowed. This rare congenital defect of the cardiac conduction system may require surgical implantation of an electrical pacemaker to stimulate the ventricles.

The normal heartbeat varies considerably in children. The younger the child, the faster the rate. For example, a heart rate of 130 beats per minute is normal for a newborn infant, but is too fast for a six-year-old child at rest without fever. On the other hand, a rate of fifty to sixty beats per minute is about normal for an athletic, well-conditioned teenager but too slow for a baby. A slow heart rate

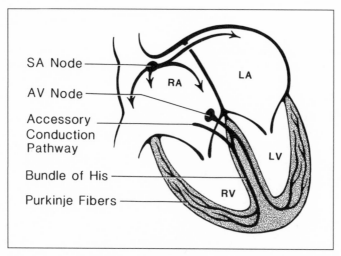

FIGURE 25

Accessory conduction pathway. This pathway exists, in addition to the normal one through the atrioventricular node (AV node and bundle of His), between the right atrium (RA) and the conduction pathway. It can cause arrhythmia. (LA = left atrium, LV = left ventricle, RV = right ventricle)

is called bradycardia. Fever, stress, and exercise or vigorous activity such as crying usually make the heart rate increase. Although the point should not be belabored, tachycardia, or abnormally rapid heartbeat, is occasionally diagnosed in children who in fact typically increase their heart rates to 160 or 170 beats per minute as a normal response to activity or to high fever.

In normal, healthy children, the rhythm of the heartbeat varies slightly when the child inhales and exhales. This is frequently observed during routine physical examinations or electrocardiograms performed for other reasons. The normal variation is called sinus arrhythmia. Because sinus arrhythmia requires no special evaluation, it should be of no concern to parents or physicians.

Extra heartbeats, also called premature or early heartbeats, are sometimes noted during a physical examination or in an electrocardiogram. They result in a mild irregularity of heart rhythm. Most children and adults experience premature beats from time to time. Usually they go unnoticed, but once in a while they are recognized and described as the heart "skipping a beat" or as a "flip-flop." Premature beats are not an indication of heart disease, especially when they go away with exercise. When the premature electrical impulse originates in the atria, the resulting beat is called a premature atrial contraction (PAC); when it originates in the ventricles, it is called a premature ventricular contraction (PVC). Mild irregularity of heartbeat, such as PACs or PVCs, usually requires no treatment at all.

Tachycardia

The most common irregularity of the heartbeat, one that does require further evaluation and often treatment, is tachycardia, an abnormally rapid heartbeat. In this condition, the heart rate abruptly increases from normal to more than 220 beats per minute. An episode may last seconds or minutes. It may even persist for hours, in which case treatment is necessary.

If your child has paroxysmal atrial tachycardia (PAT), you probably remember being alarmed the first time it occurred. Your child felt uncomfortable, weak, and probably dizzy. It should be reassuring for you to know that the heart will not suddenly stop beating, nor will the tachycardia ordinarily last the many hours necessary to cause severe illness. This type of tachycardia can be effectively treated with medication or a mild electrical shock called cardioversion.

PAT does *not* indicate that serious heart disease is present. If the episodes repeat themselves, there may be some simple things your child can do to stop the tachycardia, such as blowing up a balloon, applying cold water to his or her face, massaging the major arteries, coughing, or vomiting. The practice of putting pressure on the eyeballs is not advisable because it can cause serious damage to the eye.

If the tachycardia persists for longer than twenty or thirty minutes, your child should be taken to a physician or an emergency room for treatment. Short bursts of PAT occurring less often than once or twice a month usually do not warrant daily medication.

Most tachycardias associated with very rapid heartbeat that cannot be easily terminated by simple maneuvers can be managed by drug therapy. The medication that your doctor chooses depends on its effect on both the normal and abnormal specialized conduction tissue and its effect on the ability of the heart to contract. Some drugs slow conduction to the normal AV node but enhance conduction through accessory tissue. Some do just the opposite. There are medications that improve the heart's ability to contract and others that depress it. The exact type of arrhythmia must be defined and the drug's side effects considered before a medication is prescribed. On occasion, two or more medications may be required to control the problem.

In rare cases—when the tachycardia is life-threatening or incapacitating and medication cannot control it—surgery is necessary. The abnormal conduction tissue is cut. This highly specialized open-heart operation is performed at several institutions in the United States. Although it may be inconvenient to travel to one of these medical centers, the results of the operation are usually rewarding.

The presence of accessory specialized conduction tissue characteristic of PAT may be recognized in an electrocardiogram by a pattern called Wolff-Parkinson-White syndrome. Abnormal atrioventricular conduction of the electrical impulse caused by accessory tissue, although bothersome, is not particularly dangerous. Most children with either PAT or supraventricular tachycardia (SVT) can be effectively treated with medication. Again, specialized surgery to cut the accessory tissue is necessary only when medication is unsuccessful in controlling the arrhythmia.

Ventricular tachycardia, an abnormally fast heartbeat originating in the ventricles, is rare in children. When it occurs it indicates a potentially serious problem and is often associated with an abnormality of heart muscle or conduction tissue. Your physician can distinguish ventricular tachycardia from the much more common supraventricular type.

Bradycardia

Abnormally slow heartbeat is less common than tachycardia. The condition is called bradycardia and it may be present at birth or develop during childhood. In children, bradycardia is usually caused by damage to the natural pacemaker site, the SA node, that occurs during open-heart surgery or viral infection of the heart. This is called sick-sinus syndrome. It may be associated now and then with

PAT. Bradycardia may also be caused by the inability to transmit an impulse from the atrium to the ventricle, a condition called heart block because the impulse is blocked from making its way to the ventricle.

When bradycardia is detected prior to or shortly after birth, a congenital, complete heart block is usually the cause. This rare condition that occurs in one of every twenty thousand live births is probably due to failure of fusion of the AV node with the bundle of His. Complete heart block may be associated with other defects in the heart's structure or may be present as an isolated defect. As a result, normal conduction of the electrical impulse originating in the SA node cannot travel into the ventricles and the heart rate is extremely slow, ranging from thirty-five to sixty beats per minute.

Complete heart block may develop later in childhood. It could result from inflammatory diseases of the heart or from a cardiac operation if the tissue around the AV node has been inadvertently damaged. Heart block can also run in families. If your child is affected, the major danger is that he or she may have black-out spells.

Some children may need to have a permanent pacemaker inserted if they have congenital heart block or acquired heart block following surgical correction of congenital heart disease. In the latter case, the heart block is usually noticeable a few days after the operation. In rare cases, it appears months or years later. Any child who experiences a black-out spell following open-heart surgery should be carefully evaluated to find out if the spell was caused by heart block.

Insertion of a permanent pacemaker is a relatively easy, low-risk surgical procedure that is performed at many medical centers throughout the country. Pacemakers are virtually trouble-free, easily maintained, and last for several years before the battery must be changed. With very mild inconvenience, they allow the wearer to live a fairly normal life.

The electrocardiogram, one of the most important diagnostic tests ever developed, is often used to detect irregular heartbeat (see chapter 2). Over the past 40 years, the EKG has hardly changed. It is used to assess three aspects of the heart: (1) its rate, rhythm, and conduction pathways; (2) the size of its chambers; and (3) the adequacy of blood flow to the heart muscle. In this chapter, we will discuss only the use of the EKG to detect irregularities of the heartbeat.

The electrocardiogram is a simple method of diagnosing an irregularity of the beat, for it records the successive activation of the atria and ventricles. The heartbeat can easily be counted and the irregularities observed. Most people who have visited a hospital or watched hospital-based television shows have seen the monitor screen used to check the heart rate.

When cardiac conduction is abnormal, the pattern recorded by the electrocardiogram is altered. One previously mentioned example is that of abnormal atrioventricular conduction through accessory conduction, which is often associated with Wolff-Parkinson-White syndrome on an electrocardiogram.

Detecting a Bad Beat

If your child has an arrhythmia, he or she does not experience it all the time. Such irregularities tend to be episodic and may be induced by vigorous exertion. To determine the frequency of irregular heartbeat, a technique called twenty-four hour continuous electrocardiograph monitoring records the EKG on a small tape recorder the size of a portable radio or purse. The monitor, worn for a day or two at a time, is attached to EKG wires. Every heartbeat during that time is recorded. You and your child will be asked to keep a log of activities and symptoms experienced during this period so that they can be correlated with the EKG pattern. For example, if your child experienced several seconds of heart "flutter" and dizziness at 2:15 PM and the EKG shows PAT at the same, a diagnosis is established. Continuous monitoring has dramatically advanced our ability to detect irregular heartbeat that occurs during normal activity and sleep.

Exercise is known to set off arrhythmia in some cases. Your doctor may use stress testing on a bicycle or treadmill (see chapter 2) to reproduce symptoms characteristic of irregular heartbeat. Also, stress testing is an important way to be sure that premature beats, or extrasystoles, are not the result of cardiac disease.

If your doctor considers the problem to be potentially dangerous or if it is unresponsive to treatment with medicine, an electrophysiological (EP) study is carried out. This is a specialized type of cardiac catheterization. Several catheters are inserted to study the conduction system of the heart. An arrhythmia may be induced so that the cardiac response to medication can be investigated. An EP study has essentially the same risk as cardiac catheterization. The potential benefit to your child outweighs the small risk involved.

Until very recently, detection and analysis of irregular heartbeat before birth were very difficult; attempts to record an EKG of a fetus were generally unsuccessful. During a routine examination of a pregnant woman, a physician may by chance discover abnormalities of the fetal heart rate or rhythm. It used to be impossible to characterize the types of arrhythmia and to determine whether treatment was required; now echocardiography of the fetal heart, a noninvasive and safe procedure for both the woman and the fetus, can detect and identify the characteristics of irregular heartbeat. In addition, a view of the structures of the heart is provided that can determine whether heart disease is present. Such a study is done by pediatric cardiologists with specialized training and knowledge.

Chapter 7
CARDIAC
SURGERY

Erica is a seven-year-old delight with a smile so broad it nearly reaches her ears. She has beaten the odds over and over, and she will have to beat them again if she is to survive into adulthood. She was a blue baby. When Erica was just two days old, her parents took her to a children's hospital, where she was diagnosed with complex heart disease. Among other things, she has a single atrium and ventricle. She was "fading fast" when she was referred to a university hospital. Erica underwent emergency heart surgery.

"Erica wouldn't have survived without surgery," her mother said. "She had so many problems, and she was so swollen. We met with the surgeon and he told us that she had only a 40 percent chance of surviving the surgery and that it would be difficult to wean her from the heart-lung machine. One of the hardest things for us is that we didn't know what questions to ask."

"There was a feeling of total helplessness, that we didn't really have an option," said Erica's father. "We did a lot of thinking about whether to have the surgery done or let nature take its course. What kind of life would she have if the surgery were successful? Would she be a vegetable? We were told that she would be able to enjoy life if she survived, but that she probably wouldn't have a normal or long life. The surgeon said 'It's your decision.'"

Erica made it through surgery, but her parents were advised afterward that she had only a 10 percent chance of surviving until her first birthday. When she was six months old she had surgery again. This time a shunt was inserted to aid her circulation. At age four and again at five she had a balloon angioplasty. Erica was one of the first patients to undergo this experimental procedure. The second was an unqualified success. Doctors were able to open her pulmonary valve, inaccessible to surgeons, with the aid of

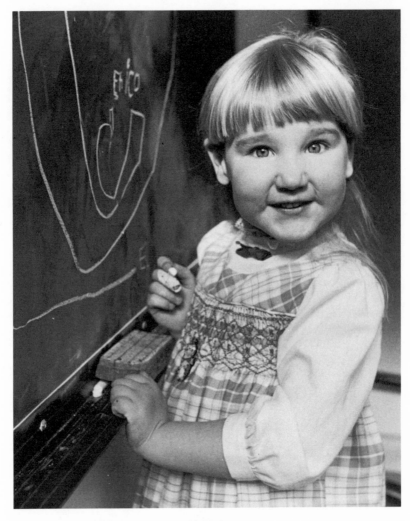

FIGURE 26

Erica at age four.

a balloon-tipped catheter. As her mother observed, "She went in blue in the morning and came out pink at night."

Today Erica is "doing very well," according to her parents, but they know that further surgery is in store for her. Because many of her internal organs are reversed, she is not a good candidate for a dramatic step that might offer her the prospect of a long life—a heart-lung transplant. Her parents try to be realistic, but they have not given up hope. After all, medical science is never without new developments, and Erica is accustomed to taking advantage of them.

Heart operations are so common these days that we tend to forget that modern cardiac surgery is only a half-century old. The surgeon who performed the first heart operation was Dr. Robert E. Gross of Boston Children's Hospital. On August 26, 1938, he and his surgical team successfully closed the patent ductus arteriosus of a seven-year-old girl. This fetal remnant of communication between the aorta and the pulmonary trunk normally closes by itself within twenty-four hours of birth. The operation was recommended by the child's cardiologist, Dr. John Hubbard.

Hubbard's contribution to this milestone of surgery is important because it helps to underscore the relationship between the cardiologist and the cardiac surgeon in the care of children with heart disease. The cardiologist establishes the correct diagnosis, decides whether surgery is necessary, and determines the opportune time for it. The surgeon studies the clinical data obtained by the cardiologist during the examination and sometimes suggests alternative approaches to solving the problem. If the surgeon concurs that surgery is necessary and can be done at an acceptable risk, surgery is recommended. In general, care of the patient during the initial postoperative period is the responsibility of the surgeon, long-term follow-up that of the cardiologist. Thus, a close working relationship exists between the cardiologist and surgeon, which helps to facilitate the best care possible. Both clearly understand their respective role and responsibility in treating the patient.

Gross and Hubbard's contribution heralded unprecedented advances in treating children with heart disease. In 1944, for example, Dr. Helen Taussig, a pediatrician in charge of the heart clinic at Johns Hopkins University, urged surgeon Dr. Alfred Blalock to perform an operation that resulted in a major improvement in the outlook for children with tetralogy of Fallot, the most common form of cyanotic congenital heart disease (see chapter 4). This operation, called palliative shunt procedure, did not actually correct the underlying heart defects, but it did allow children to live many more years on average than they otherwise would have.

It was not until 1953 that total correction of cardiac defects became possible, thanks to the pioneering work of Drs. Henry Gibbons, C. Walton Lillehei, and others involved in the development of the heart-lung bypass procedure. This procedure made it possible for circulation to be sustained during surgery. Advances in open-heart surgery since 1953 have been astounding. Today, most congenital heart defects are repaired during infancy with a technique that, in a sense, puts the baby in a state of suspended animation by dramatically lowering body temperature.

Selecting a Heart Surgeon

You have an obligation to see that your child receives the best possible medical care. But how can you decide who to have operate on your child's heart? As lay people, you have to place your trust in a medical specialist, that is, in your child's primary care physician, usually a pediatrician or family practitioner. Because family practitioners and pediatricians care for other children with heart problems, they invariably have established a referral relationship with a pediatric cardiologist they trust and respect.

Your child's cardiologist is the most appropriate physician to recommend a heart surgeon for the particular problem that your child has. As already mentioned, the cardiologist has a close working relationship with a cardiac surgical team. The cardiologist is in the best position to monitor surgical performance, keep abreast of developments in the field, and regularly confer with colleagues about the most reliable and advanced therapeutic and surgical techniques. It is obvious that pediatric cardiology and cardiovascular surgery for children are closely related fields, and no other medical specialist is likely to be as knowledgeable about these fields as your child's cardiologist. Remember that the first obligation of the cardiologist is to you and your child, not to a particular surgeon or surgical team. Ultimately the decision is yours. However, your cardiologist will recommend only an experienced surgeon who has a clear record of acceptable results. And, although friends' and relatives' advice about surgeons may be well intentioned, it will more than likely be confusing. You, in consultation with your child's doctor, are in a much better position to make such a decision.

Seeking a Second Opinion

If you do have doubts about a surgical procedure or surgical team recommended by your cardiologist, consider seeking a second opinion from another pediatric cardiologist. This request should not offend your child's cardiologist, and he or she can help with the necessary arrangements.

Bear in mind that whichever surgeon you choose, he or she has received the rigorous and intensive training essential for certification to perform such surgery. Following completion of the prescribed surgical training, usually six or seven years beyond completion of medical school, surgeons must pass written and oral examinations to test their competency. Your child's surgeon should be certified by the American Board of Thoracic Surgery. Moreover, surgeons are becoming increasingly specialized. For years cardiovascular surgeons have been trained to correct congenital and acquired defects of the heart in both adults and children. However, there is a trend in the United States for the most complex cardiac surgical procedures in infants to be done by cardiothoracic surgeons who have subspecialized in the care of such patients.

It is normal when one of us or a loved one is seriously ill to think that the farther away from home we go for medical care the better the care we will receive. This is simply not true in most cases. Medicine and health care are tightly regulated in the United States so that a high standard of competence is normally maintained. Your child's cardiologist will probably recommend the best possible surgeon at a facility that is closest to your home. It is rarely necessary to go halfway across the country to receive good care.

The Hospital Stay

It is hardly reasonable for you to expect that you will not be nervous when the time comes for your child to undergo heart surgery. What parent would not be anxious given the uncertainty and risk of a major complication and even death? By informing yourself as much as possible about the nature of the problem, the surgery being performed, and the risks involved, you may be better able to control that anxiety. Medical and hospital staff can help you in this respect, and you should not hesitate to call on them.

The pediatric cardiologist responsible for your child will already have explained why surgery is recommended at this time. Sometimes arrangements are made for you to talk with the surgeon before your child is admitted to the hospital. The surgeon will sit down with you and go over the details of the procedure, including the possible complications. This is not only an ethical but also a legal requirement.

The cardiology and surgical teams want you to understand what is to be done. They will also discuss it with your child if he or she is old enough or able to comprehend why an operation is important. Care is taken so that your child will not become frightened, but it is certainly not fair to be dishonest. It is helpful for a nurse clinician, a member of the surgical team, to take you and your child to the entrance of the operating room and the pediatric intensive care unit the day before surgery. If your child is young, the nurse clinician may try to explain the operation by demonstrating on a doll or teddy bear. Your child may want to take the toy into the operating room on the day of the surgery. When he or she wakes up after the operation, the doll or teddy bear will have bandages on its chest too.

The Recovery Room

You may be concerned about being kept away from your child during the immediate postoperative period. This separation enables the medical staff to deliver the constant care needed at this critical time, without being interrupted. Besides, your child will still be partially asleep from anesthesia and sedation. To allay undue fear, you may request to see your child in the intensive care unit for a few minutes following the operation. After that it is best for you to be available but not to request exceptions from established visiting policy.

Usually each day following surgery is a little better. Your child is recovering. As the critical postoperative phase passes, you can visit him or her more often. By the time your child really needs to have

you on hand, he or she is ready to be transferred from the intensive
care unit into the regular pediatric ward or intermediate care unit,
often a matter of several days after the operation. Now your anxiety
will begin to subside.

Heart operations in children can require a few days to several
weeks of hospitalization, depending on the seriousness of the procedure, the condition of the child, and whether complications arise.
Occasionally, the child will recover so slowly that prolonged
hospitalization is necessary, but this is the exception.

When it is time for your child to be discharged, hospital nurses
will explain how and when to administer any medications that are
prescribed, and the cardiologist or surgeon will arrange for appropriate follow-up care.

Kids that have a heart defect
are just like other kids. Jason is
an active and curious fellow
and a good patient, his doctor
says.

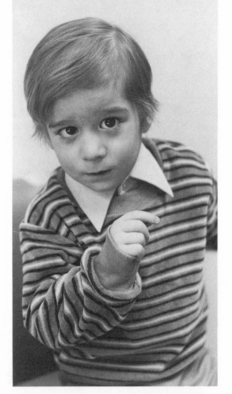

Brothers and sisters can help to
make life easier for a child with
a heart defect. Here Jason (left)
and his brother wait for the
doctor.

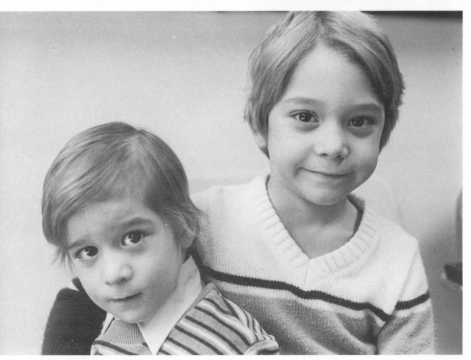

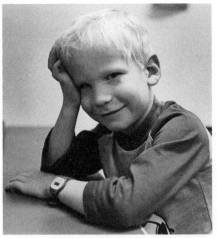

Michael was born with a heart defect that was repaired by surgery. He is an active and sports-minded young man, with a special interest in wrestling.

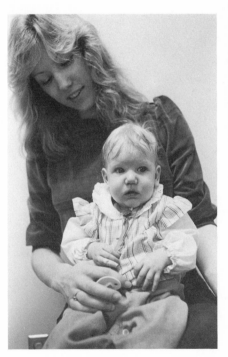

Michael likes to be read to by his father. Parents play a vital role in their child's development and ability to cope with the medical problems asociated with a heart defect.

Terese was born with her major heart vessels in the wrong places. The outlook for patients like Terese after surgery is very good.

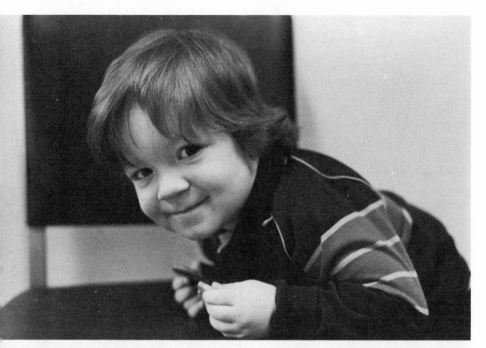

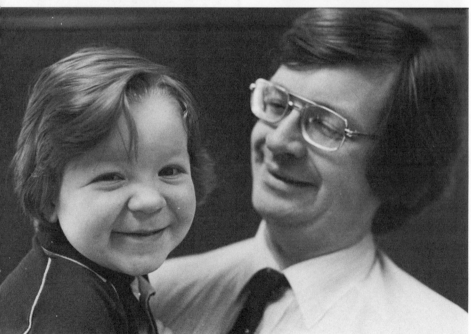

Martin had a heart defect that was corrected by an operation. Now he likes to go fishing with his father.

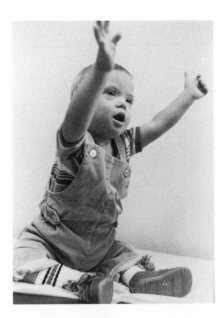

Filling the special needs of a child with a heart defect does not go unrewarded. Zachary is a joy to his parents.

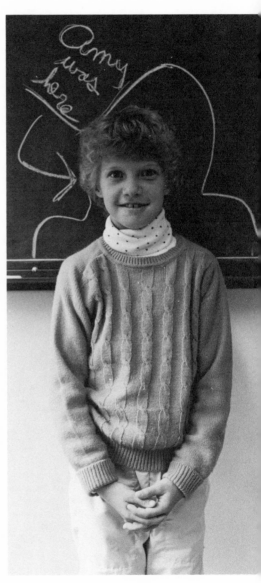

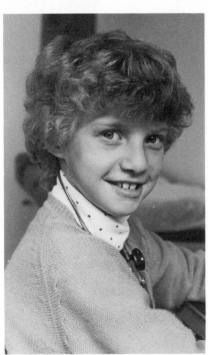

Amy had a heart operation 10 years ago. Her dream is to become a flight attendant.

Chapter 8
COPING WITH A
GROWING CHILD

Erica, *the seven year old you met at the beginning of chapter 7, came home from school one day and told her mother that her classmates were asking about her purple lips. Naturally she asked her mother why she had purple lips.*

"In my infinite wisdom, I said 'Because God made them that way,'" her mother recalled. Undeterred, Erica decided on a course of action. "Let's ask God for a different color," she said.

Once Erica was with her mother in a grocery store and a woman in the checkout line remarked that Erica looked cold. "I suppose I should have told her that Erica wasn't cold and explained why she had that bluish cast," she said.

Erica's parents admit that she does not really understand her situation. "We're not attempting to hide anything from her," her father said. "Our feeling is that she should be told when she is ready to know. Right now she is pretending everything is normal."

As parents of a child with a heart defect, you may often feel helpless—that you have little direct control over the complicated process of attending to your child's medical problem, You may find yourselves in awkward situations. Yet you do play a vital role in your child's development and ability to cope with his or her medical problems.

Even if your child has a severe problem, he or she spends much less time in a doctor's office or hospital than at home or in school. As parents, you decide what kind of environment your child will live in. Your child's physician may offer suggestions in this regard, but the final decisions are yours. There is no substitute for good supportive care while your child is at home, in school, or playing with friends.

How to Care for Your Infant

No sooner had her parents brought Erica home from the hospital after her emergency surgery than they were confronted with a problem common in infants with congenital heart disease. Erica could not keep food down. In addition to her heart malformation, she was missing the ring of muscles that prevents food in the stomach from reentering the esophagus.

"We tried mixing rice cereal with her milk to make it heavier, and she was able to keep that down a little better," Erica's mother said. "When we started her on solid food she had trouble again, but everything changed when she was about a year and a half. The doctor says she learned to control it."

"When she was about four she started complaining about a burning feeling in her stomach, especially when she was upset," her mother said. "We give her antacid and that seems to take care of the problem."

Erica is a picky eater, but "she can get through a meal if there's a cookie at the end of it," her father said.

Even if you have experience in caring for infants, the prospect of caring for a baby with a heart defect can be frightening. You not only feel the usual sense of responsibility but also realize that you are dealing with a condition that is often unpredictable and occasionally even deadly.

Of course, we all have older relatives or neighbors who have a "heart condition." We know that adults with coronary artery disease may have to limit their activities, follow special diets, and alter their habits to lower their risk of heart attack. Bear in mind, however, that heart disease among the very young and the elderly cannot be compared. The same "rules" do not apply.

An infant with a congenital heart defect, for example, is born with a malformed heart, but most such infants are otherwise vigorous and healthy. The fact is that the young, with rare exception, do not have heart "attacks." Many infants with congenital heart disease require no special care other than periodic visits to the cardiologist. Their feeding routine is the same as for other babies. They receive their immunizations at the usually prescribed time, and their activity is not restricted, which is just as well since restricting them is practically impossible.

Crying does not hurt a baby. During the first several months of infancy, crying often means that your baby is wet or hungry. As your baby approaches one year, he or she may register discontent by crying for being put to bed or left alone. With age, there is less reason to pacify your child unless there is an obvious problem. Regardless of your child's age, you should treat him or her as normal. The fact that he or she has a heart defect will usually require minimal modification, if any, of child-rearing practices.

However, if your baby has a serious congenital heart disease, you will most likely have to make modifications. For example, it may be necessary to alter feeding practices until he or she is old enough to have corrective surgery. After surgery, your child is not likely to have symptoms related to heart disease.

If your infant is discharged from the hospital with chronic but controlled congestive heart failure, he or she will not be able to feed or suck as vigorously as a healthy baby. More time will probably be required for your baby to take enough formula or breast milk to be satisfied. On occasion, more frequent feedings and smaller amounts may be necessary. Special "preemie" nipples make it easier for your baby to suck. Do not worry; we have found that parents often do a better job with this careful feeding than do hospital nurses, who are usually pressed for time. It requires only a little extra patience to make sure that your baby takes enough nourishment to grow.

If your infant has congestive heart failure from a congenital defect, medicines may help by making the heart beat more vigorously or by removing excessive fluid that is burdensome to the cardiovascular system. In the former instance, Lanoxin is often prescribed, and in the latter, a diuretic. These medications are prepared in such a way that they are easy for you to administer in the proper concentration, usually with a dropper. The use of small syringes to orally administer the medicines, a common practice on pediatric wards, is not really necessary. If your infant spits up some of the medication, do not try to guess the amount and make up the difference. It is better for your baby to miss a full dose than to be overdosed.

Your doctor will assess your baby's growth and development during the periodic check-ups. You should know that congenital heart disease, even when cyanosis or "blue baby" results, does not significantly affect mental development. However, chronic congestive heart failure may slow growth somewhat, which in turn can diminish muscle development and strength. For example, an eight-month-old baby with a serious heart condition may have the will but not the strength to sit up alone. As physicians, we accept a certain degree of failure-to-thrive in an infant who is chronically ill so that surgery can be performed more safely later on.

Just when things seem to be going well, you may be advised that it is time for your toddler or preschooler to have an operation. You and your baby have made it through the trials and tribulations of infancy and now you have to face the anxiety-producing prospect of major surgery and hospitalization. It is understandable if you are nervous, but the likelihood that everything will turn out all right is very good and getting better all the time. Nonetheless, it is best to be prepared so that when the time comes you have the necessary emotional reserves to draw from.

Your Child Goes to School

Erica's parents try not to be overprotective, which is no easy task. Their overriding concern is that Erica should develop at her own pace in a normal environment at home and in school. They held her back an extra year in kindergarten. They wonder how she will do when she attends school full days, whether she will need a rest period, perhaps at home. Erica has a pleasant personality, her parents said, but she finds it difficult adjusting to new situations.

"One thing we don't want to do with Erica is put her into high-pressure situations," her mother said. "We are more concerned about how our other kids do academically. We just want her to be in a comfortable and happy environment."

Erica's father said it was difficult to convince her teachers, especially her physical education teacher, that she should not be treated differently from other kids. "We told her phy. ed. teacher that we wanted Erica to be involved," he said. "If she's tired, she'll sit down. If her stomach hurts, she should go to the nurse's office. It's important for her teachers to know enough to let her participate and not to panic. We have to explain why she won't have a heart attack in class, that what she has is not the same type of thing as a heart attack. We try to be open."

In the United States, every child has a right to public education. Congress passed Public Law 94–142 in 1975, which establishes the principle that children with handicapping or disabling conditions are entitled to free public education in the least restrictive setting. Many are better served educationally and socially in a normal school environment than in a private setting.

Children with congenital heart disease have never been restricted from attending school to the same extent as those with more observable defects, such as children with deformed or missing limbs. Even so, in the past it was not uncommon for parents of cyanotic children to be encouraged, and occasionally even required, to arrange for home-bound teachers. There was considerable fear among teachers and administrators that the child might suffer some sudden catastrophe if placed in a public school. It is true today that many cyanotic children are restricted from fully participating in physical education classes, even though such classes are rarely detrimental to their health.

Most children with congenital heart disease who are not cyanotic—who do not have a bluish cast from poorly oxygenated blood—have no visible symptoms and do not tire more easily than other children. Often it is up to parents themselves to reassure teachers and administrators that their child can participate in all normal school activities, including physical education, without restriction.

If your child is cyanotic, he or she will tire more easily than other children, usually in proportion to the degree of cyanosis present. In this situation, you should arrange a conference with the school principal or homeroom teacher to explain the condition and show supporting medical documents, if necessary. This way you and the school authorities can best decide how to handle whatever limitations may exist so that your child can reach his or her maximum level of achievement.

You should not have unreasonable expectations of the school. Most schools want to accommodate handicapped children in a way that is least disruptive to other students. For example, if it takes your child ten minutes to climb stairs to the third floor for a class and only five minutes is available between classes, you should insist that the child not be penalized for arriving a few minutes late. Likewise, it is advisable to confer with physical education instructors about any limitation of activity recommended by your child's cardiologist so that appropriate alternatives can be sought.

The Vibrant Teenage Heart

"Reminding James to take his medications three times a day is one of the biggest problems," said the mother of the fifteen-year-old boy described at the beginning of chapter 5. "It's not unusual for him to forget. It's almost as if he doesn't want to take it. I put it out on the table with water and he will walk right past it. He says he's busy, or in a hurry, or just forgets. We think it's a sign of rebelliousness—that he does it just to annoy us. I've gotten really angry with him. If something happened, I would feel responsible."

James's father added: "I would like to invent a box, a pill case with a clock, alarm, and settings. It might remind him to take his pills."

Like most parents of adolescents, you probably are tested by the rapid emotional and physical changes taking place in your child during this crucial period. Throw in a serious medical problem, and you may understandably feel overwhelmed.

As a rule, teenagers with heart disease differ little if at all from their peers in physical development. Severe congestive heart failure or profound cyanosis in childhood may lead to slower-than-normal growth or may delay somewhat the onset of puberty. We simply reassure affected children that the expected changes in their bodies will occur in time. Emotional development, however, may not be as easy to deal with, among other reasons because the process takes longer. Adolescents are often more withdrawn and less communicative than they were when they were children. Some of them spend long hours alone listening to music, frequently at decibel levels above those comfortable for adults. Others are absorbed in television or video games, or, in some instances, books.

The teenage emotional response is seen by adults as exaggerated. Teens are argumentative, "rebellious," and easily offended. To the rest of us, they appear to behave as if the world revolves around them, and when the world does not see things their way they feel misunderstood, especially by their parents. And parents, of course, are in the position of having to impose limits and restrictions that the adolescent struggles to break free of.

Adolescence is a terribly ambivalent time of life. The teenager wants the attention and support he or she got as a child, but at the same time seeks the freedom of adulthood. Since they are part child and part adult, such incongruity should not surprise us.

The self-image of a teenager is fragile and peer pressure is great.

So it is natural for the adolescent with symptomatic heart disease to feel threatened because he or she may not be able to participate in athletic events or other activities to the same extent as others. They want to prove to parents, teachers, and peers that they have no limitations. By sheer willpower they will show that they are just like their friends and classmates, if not better.

As parents, you should try to recognize and understand these feelings and attitudes. Although your teenager may deny the heart problem, he or she may actually be eager to know more about it and how it will affect the future. When your teenager is ready, the cardiologist will make a point of discussing with him or her in detail the implications of the heart abnormality. Most teenagers respond well to this approach, realizing that the physician is directing his or her attention to them as individuals with the capacity to be responsible for their own well-being.

We suggest that your teenager be accountable for taking medications, without being reminded. You will no doubt be relieved to relinquish this responsibility. If your doctor senses that you are being overprotective, he or she may give you a gentle nudging along these lines.

The cardiologist will begin to pay special attention to the level of your child's physical activity at adolescence. Most types of congenital or acquired heart disease will not limit even strenuous activity. One exception is serious aortic stenosis, a narrowing of the aortic valve. This may create a risk for developing a potentially fatal arrhythmia after exertion for a prolonged period. Surgery will probably be recommended if the degree of obstruction is severe.

Meanwhile, your adolescent must understand why limitations in physical activity are necessary and what alternatives are safer. Children rest when they are tired; adolescents may try to push themselves beyond their endurance to prove a point. Since valvular aortic stenosis is twice as common in males as in females, we urge affected boys to go out for sports that do not require prolonged exertion, such as baseball. We point out to them that 99 percent of the normal activities of adults are safe for them and that they are perfectly capable of becoming productive citizens and should not think of themselves as cardiac cripples.

Of course you want your child to enjoy life to the fullest and not to be unduly burdened by a medical disability. You can attain this goal with the cardiologist's help in preparing your teenager for adulthood.

Chapter 9

DEATH, DYING, AND GRIEVING

"**M**y husband and I knew that Justin would eventually have to have another heart operation, but we were scared when the time actually came. Even Justin knew that something was wrong. He was starting to get blue and tire out so easily. I think he wanted the operation so he could be just like other children. He wasn't as frightened as we were, maybe because we told him he would be pink and run and play like his friends. I used to feel so guilty that we told him he would be all right, but not anymore. I didn't want him to be frightened.*

Justin was only seven when he died. . . . "How have we coped? We didn't for a while. It was the saddest time of my life, worse than when my mother died. Steve, my husband, handled it differently. He wouldn't talk about it for months, but I knew he was suffering just as much. He is much better now. Two years have passed. I'm better, too, but you never get over it. The pain just lessens. It helps to know that we and Justin's doctors did all that we could. I guess it was just not meant to be."

This story, as told to a parent support group, gives only a hint of the suffering experienced by parents when they lose a child. Yet this woman was able not only to survive her child's death but to emerge with healthy emotions and with her experience in perspective.

As physicians, we are relieved to know that this woman was able to recover from the immediate pain and sorrow of her loss and to move forward in her own life. Of course, she and her husband were realistically afraid of the possibility that Justin would die before the surgery could be done. You cannot prepare for this by denying that death may be the result. But these parents did not approach their child's operation with a feeling of failure or impending doom either. They were optimistic and conveyed this optimism to Justin.

Was the expression of such optimism unfair to their seven-year-old child? No purpose would have been served by adding to the apprehension of this mentally and emotionally normal child who was capable of some understanding of death. Justin trusted his parents and willingly accepted the operation, even though he knew it was not without some risk.

The death of a child from disease has become relatively uncommon today compared with a few generations ago. We are not as well prepared for a child's death as our grandparents were. In their time, many infants or children were lost to infection or other childhood diseases. We have come so far in obstetric and pediatric medicine that we think it just cannot happen anymore. But it can, and if your child has a serious heart defect, you need to be emotionally prepared for this possibility. You must also prepare your child if he or she is old enough to have some understanding of death.

A Child's Understanding of Death

You may wonder at what age children understand the meaning of death. The many studies on child development do not give an unequivocal answer to this question.

The level of a child's understanding of death is dependent, to some degree, on his or her previous experience, such as the death of a relative or family member. Surely a four-year-old child living in a starving African country has a better understanding of death than a typical American child of the same age. Likewise, a chronically ill child who has been repeatedly hospitalized in a large medical center may be more aware of death than a healthy child.

Comprehension of the finality of death depends on your child's age as well as his or her experience. Your attitude about death, especially the way you handle the deaths of relatives and close friends, strongly influences the way your child will feel when confronted with this reality.

From the age of seven years, most children have a sufficient understanding of death to justify honest answers to their questions. Younger children also deserve honest answers but perhaps with less detail. You know that children are incredibly egocentric; they believe that they are somehow responsible for everything that happens around them. They may feel they are being punished for their own transgressions. For this reason, children must be made to understand that they are not to blame for the death of a sibling or parent (or for their own illness). They need to know that everyone involved in the care of their deceased loved one did all they could to save his or her life. And young children should be reassured that other family members are not in danger of dying soon.

The Grieving Process

Grieving is a normal and necessary expression to ensure that the pain of loss does not cripple the survivors. Mourning serves three purposes: it helps break ties with the deceased person; it allows formation of new ties to replace those with the deceased; and it helps resolve feelings of guilt, anger, and ambivalence precipitated by the death of a loved one.

The noted psychologist and author Elizabeth Kubler-Ross has found that the grieving process involves several very natural stages. The first is overwhelming bewilderment or denial. We are unprepared to cope with the sudden finality of death. Parents of a deceased child may feel the loss more keenly than others. They brought the child into the world, nurtured and protected it, and now the child is gone forever. They tell themselves "It can't be true!" Developing and drawing from the immense emotional reserves necessary to deal with the death of a child takes time. Parents must be willing to grant themselves that time. At first, they want to believe that there has been some mistake. Viewing, holding, and even talking to the dead child is often necessary for parents before they fully realize that their child is dead.

The denial stage is often followed by guilt. It is not uncommon for guilt to be overwhelming and replaced with anger. The anger is initially unfocused but soon can be directed at someone: at God, at the other parent, at medical staff. Sometimes the "safest" outlet for parental anger is the physician most involved in the care of the child. This is usually not the surgeon, who may be seen as merely an instrument, but the cardiologist. After all, the cardiologist recommended or "talked the parents into" the operation.

In these instances, anger directed at the attending physician lessens with the passing of time and with the parents' acceptance that they themselves knew the risks of the operation and agreed to it. Parents must realize that they were powerless, in effect, to act or decide in any way other than the way they did. They sought the medical attention that was needed for their child. They followed the recommendation of their child's doctor. There was no way for them to know that, despite the best efforts of the medical staff, their child was going to die.

Preparation for the possibility of death helps. As physicians, we sense on occasion that parents are totally denying this possibility before the child enters surgery. Frequently we point out to them that they are acting on the best advice available to give their child a chance for life or an improved quality of life, but that even modern medicine cannot give guarantees. If we could see the future, we might choose a different course of action. Because we cannot, we base our decisions and recommendations on the best information we have.

Once the recommendation is made to continue treatment or perform surgery, and is accepted by the parents, we cannot look back. Parents who have unrealistic or morbid fears before the operation need to be counseled, but no cardiologist or surgeon will proceed with treatment without the parents willingly granting their consent. Communication with the parents throughout the course of the child's care helps to prepare them for any eventuality, even death.

If death is the outcome, the pain of loss must be experienced. Medication to dull feelings or sublimate the grief should be avoided. Drugs or alcohol only delay the process of dealing with death. Acceptance is essential before recovery from the death of a child can occur.

Of course, parents do not really get over the death or forget about their child. Even newborn babies who die after only a few days are forever a part of the life of a parent. But parents must allow themselves time to grieve and understand that time heals emotional wounds just as it does physical wounds. Some parents require more time to move through the various stages of grief than others. They must realize this and give each other the necessary time. They should avoid making hasty decisions about their child's belongings or about moving.

During the first weeks or months after the death of a child, it is important for parents to let their close friends and relatives know how they feel. There is no substitute for the support friends and family can offer. Within three to four weeks most parents have reached a point in mourning at which they are able to think rationally about the events surrounding the death of their child. They may be able to think about the implications of the death for their family, especially if they are thinking about having more children.

If an autopsy was performed, they are ready to hear the results. A conference with the physician who cared for their child should be arranged. This meeting can be invaluable for getting answers to nagging questions and putting things into perspective. Any lingering anger toward the physician needs to be resolved. Most physicians who care for children with major medical problems understand and do not resent this anger so long as it does not persist. Bitterness about the past can only harm all concerned.

After several months many parents choose to participate in a support group (see Appendix D). It helps to be around others who have shared the same or a similar experience. Some parents in the group may be having to deal with crucial decisions concerning a child currently undergoing treatment. In our experience, one woman who lost her two-year-old daughter served as a volunteer in a cardiac clinic, and her husband requested the opportunity to talk with their child's physician over a beer. He simply wanted to relate his feelings of grief and be reassured that it was all right that he periodically drove back to the hospital to be close to the place where his child had died.

Parents who are considering having more children should wait a year or two. A new baby cannot replace the dead child, and it takes a while for parents to accept another child as an individual in its own right and not as a substitute for the one they lost. Death is inseparable from life, and after a time parents will begin to cherish the memories of their child, not without pain, but in a way that is altogether human and life-affirming.

Chapter 10
NEW HORIZONS IN PREVENTION AND RESEARCH

Regardless of whether your child has a heart problem, you should help him or her develop healthy habits to lower the risk of cardiovascular disease occurring in adulthood. Conditions such as angina, myocardial infarction or heart attack, high blood pressure, and stroke result from degenerative processes during aging.

If this is true—and studies show that these processes do take place—what can be done? Research has shown that people who follow certain health habits can slow the rate of these potentially dangerous changes. Each of us can do things right now to improve our health and possibly increase our life span. As cardiologists, we believe these health habits are so important that parents should do their utmost to instill them in their children at an early age.

The health habits we wish to promote are intended to slow the process of atherosclerosis (hardening of the arteries). Atherosclerosis is a serious problem because the arteries become narrowed, restricting blood flow to vital organs such as the heart, brain, and kidneys. This narrowing can lead to high blood pressure, heart attack, and stroke. If we could prevent or delay these diseases, the effort would be worthwhile.

Hardening of the arteries begins in childhood and progresses during adolescence and young adulthood, even though serious problems do not occur until middle age. Clearly, then, efforts to prevent or retard this process should be directed at children since substantial and potentially irreversible damage may already exist by the third or fourth decade of life, before any symptoms are present.

The cause of atherosclerosis remains unknown, but several factors increase the risk of developing the disease. These factors have been demonstrated in adults through numerous and detailed studies in cardiovascular epidemiology. Whether the risk factors in adults influence the atherosclerotic process in children has not been firmly established. Because of the toll atherosclerotic disease extracts in terms of disability and premature death, efforts to prevent this disease are of paramount importance. The American Heart Association believes that modification of six adult risk factors in children may lead to the establishment of good habits that will extend into adulthood and reduce the risk of developing atherosclerosis (see Appendix E).

Keeping Cholesterol under Control

Cholesterol is a type of fat that circulates in the blood. It is also found in the walls of arteries that are affected by atherosclerosis. Certain foods we eat, such as eggs, butter, and fatty red meat, are rich in cholesterol.

In countries where diet contains little cholesterol, the amount of atherosclerosis is low, and in countries where the diet is high in cholesterol, the incidence of atherosclerosis is high. There is no definitive proof that a decrease in the amount of cholesterol in the blood will have an effect in later life. Nevertheless, we believe that a modest change in your child's diet, mainly a reduction of cholesterol-rich food, may be beneficial over his or her lifetime.

Red meat, eggs, and dairy products can be replaced with foods such as fish, poultry, fruits, vegetables, and cereals. These are all low in cholesterol. Margarine should be used instead of butter. Ice milk should replace ice cream. Skim milk or milk with 1 or 2 percent butterfat should be used instead of whole milk. Food with high fat content such as sausage, luncheon meat, and pastries should be restricted in your child's diet.

Eating habits and food preferences are established in early childhood. Modifications can best be achieved through altering your entire family's eating habits. You should set the example for your children. You should also think about improving your own health.

Trimming Down

Like Fat Albert, a cartoon character on a Saturday morning television show, many children are overweight. That in itself is not necessarily dangerous. Being overweight is a less clearly defined risk factor for the development of atherosclerosis, but it is associated with high blood pressure and high cholesterol levels, both of which are associated with an increased incidence of atherosclerosis of the coronary arteries that supply blood to the heart.

People who are 20 percent or more overweight are considered obese. Many obese children become obese adults. The cause of obesity in children is unknown but is believed to result from consuming more calories than are used. Obesity is more likely to develop in children because of the rapid weight gain that normally occurs while children grow. Obesity is also more likely when one or both of a child's parents are obese or when parents use food to control behavior in an infant or child, such as the practice of rewarding a child with sweets. Weight control or weight reduction will reduce most other risk factors for atherosclerosis.

Efforts should be made to curtail obesity. Such efforts must be directed at families because obesity tends to be "a family affair." If obesity or a tendency toward being overweight is a problem in your family, seek help from your physician or through a recommended weight control program. Avoid fad or crash diets. As a well-known nutritionist once said, "Diet fads are for the birds if you don't like birds." We want you not only to achieve weight control but also to develop satisfactory eating habits for your entire family. Of course, regular exercise is an essential ingredient in any program designed to maintain weight because it has a direct bearing on the number of calories consumed.

In 1985, a National Institutes of Health panel studying the health implications of obesity concluded that children, as well as adults, should reduce if they are overweight. It went on to say that, although obese children are at risk for being obese as adults, most overweight children grow up to be of normal weight. Therefore, excessive zeal or worry on the part of parents toward their overweight child is not advisable.

In assessing obesity as a risk factor in heart disease, however, the NIH panel declared obesity a disease and ranked it along with smoking and high blood pressure as a major risk factor in cardiovascular disease.

Staying off Tobacco Road

On the subject of smoking, it is best to let the facts speak for themselves. Cigarette smoking is the single most preventable cause of heart and blood vessel disease, chronic lung disease, and cancer. The effect of cigarette smoking on the risk of developing cardiovascular disease is independent of other risk factors. The risk posed by cigarette smoking is dramatically increased if other factors such as high blood pressure or elevated cholesterol level are also present.

A Gallup Poll taken in 1985 reported that 35 percent of adults in the United States had smoked cigarettes during the week before being interviewed. That percentage, which had declined by 10 percent since the surgeon general's 1964 report linking cigarette smoking and serious illness, equaled the lowest figure since Gallup began conducting audits in 1944. In the 1985 report, 38 percent of respondents aged eighteen to twenty-nine years said they smoked cigarettes.

Cigarette smoking often begins early in adolescence, when youngsters are only twelve to fourteen years old and the pattern is well established in many seventeen and eighteen year olds. The incidence of teenage smoking increased in the 1970s but recently has been declining, perhaps because of widespread efforts to warn teenagers of the dangers involved. Even though most teens are now aware of the health risks, smoking remains a problem.

A number of things could cause a teenager to begin smoking cigarettes, including peer pressure, parental example, advertisements that suggest smoking is manly or glamorous, rebelliousness, and a feeling of personal failure. You can set an example for your child by not smoking. Programs are being developed by the American Heart Association, American Lung Association, and American Cancer Society to educate children about the health risks and to help teenagers break the habit. These are valuable resources for both you and your child if smoking is a problem.

Keeping in Shape

Regular exercise may not prevent atherosclerosis, but it may protect against coronary heart disease and improve the likelihood of survival following a heart attack. Exercise does have beneficial effects.

It makes the heart and blood vessels work more efficiently. It also makes people feel better. Since exercise increases the number of calories burned, it is valuable in helping your child lose or maintain weight. Exercise also reduces tension and stress. Life is full of stress, even for children.

Your child should develop the habit of regular exercise so that physical activity continues into adult life. Most children are active and like to run and play. In our society, children are often attracted to competitive sports such as baseball, basketball, football, hockey, and gymnastics, but after high school or college, participation in these sports markedly decreases. Recreational sports such as golf, tennis, swimming, and jogging can be enjoyed throughout life. As a parent, you should encourage your child to develop interests in such activities. You may want to emphasize recreational activities rather than highly organized competitive activities.

Dealing with High Blood Pressure

As adults, we are used to having our blood pressure checked to see if it is elevated. High blood pressure, whether passing or permanent, is known to contribute to atherosclerosis. The risk of having high blood pressure is greater when other risk factors are also present.

In children, the risk from high blood pressure is not fully known. Only about 10 percent of children with high blood pressure develop sustained high blood pressure as adults. According to the American Heart Association about sixty million American adults have high blood pressure or are being treated for hypertension. About 2.7 million children ages six through seventeen have high blood pressure when their readings are adjusted for their age. Black Americans have moderate or severe hypertension two to three times as often as whites.

Children three years old and older should have their blood pressure measured by their doctor at each routine examination. Although blood pressure of children is being measured more frequently these days, it is still neglected during many physical examinations. If your child's blood pressure is not taken during an examination, be sure to ask why. Elevated blood pressure over several measurements indicates an abnormal condition. If this is the case, further diagnostic tests should be performed.

You can help your child by several relatively simple steps. For example, you can help him or her maintain a normal weight and avoid excessive intake of salt. People who eat a lot of salt—either presalted food or food they load up with salt—are more likely to have high blood pressure. The diet of children and adolescents typically contains food with a lot of salt such as soups, hot dogs, luncheon meat, crackers, chips, french fries, pizza, and hamburgers.

It can be quite difficult to reduce or eliminate some of these foods from your child's diet, but you can decrease how often you prepare and serve them with some planning. Other foods, such as fresh fruit, should be substituted as snacks. Using a salt shaker should be discouraged. Help your child and yourselves by making these diet changes for the whole family.

Some families have a history of heart disease and members sometimes die of heart attack or stroke at a comparatively young age. Children from such families are at a greater risk of developing heart disease themselves. Genetic makeup cannot be changed, so the program of prevention described in Appendix E should be followed carefully to ensure that these children are not increasing their risk.

Important Advances in Research

Every year we learn more about the heart and heart disease, thanks to the work being done at medical research centers in the United States, Canada, and overseas. Some of the research is focused on basic factors that influence the heart, such as the structure of genes and the proteins they manufacture. Other research is directed toward finding the best treatment for a particular heart problem or the effect of diet on the development of cardiovascular disease.

Sometimes it may take twenty years or more from the time someone has an idea to the point where it has been refined sufficiently to benefit a patient. We are fortunate that the National Institutes of Health and voluntary health organizations such as the American Heart Association help to fund scientific investigators so that they can do their work without the demand for "instant payoff." Indeed, open-heart surgery, which we take for granted today, was once an experimental procedure funded by these very organizations. Many experiments being done today will probably make a major difference in how we will treat heart disease in a decade or two.

As a result of research efforts, a number of new diagnostic and therapeutic methods are just beginning to become available. Also, many new medications have been developed in the past few years. Although they are initially tested in adult patients, mainly because many more adults have heart disease, these drugs are being tested in some child patients as well. The medications allow for more specific and directed treatment of arrhythmias and congestive heart failure and may eventually replace some of our current drugs.

The anti-inflammatory drug indomethacin shows promise of becoming the treatment of choice in newborn infants, often premature, whose ductus arteriosus fails to close. This fetal blood vessel that connects the pulmonary artery with the aorta normally closes within a day or two of birth. When this does not occur naturally, indomethacin can stimulate it to do so. Although this drug is not always successful and does have side effects, it is a genuine alternative to surgery. In 1985 the U. S. Food and Drug Administration approved this use of indomethacin, which is also used to treat arthritis.

One of the products of the new biotechnology is tissue plasminogen activator (TPA), which appears to dissolve blood clots in arteries and veins. A pioneering study is underway at the University of Minnesota's Heart-Lung Institute to see whether TPA helps to clear the blocked arteries of patients with certain types of angina. TPA could become an important treatment for atherosclerosis and pulmonary embolism.

Of the new diagnostic techniques that have been developed recently, perhaps the most dramatic is nuclear magnetic resonance. In this test, the patient is placed in a large and powerful magnetic field and pictures are taken. The magnetic field creates slight disturbances in the molecules that make up heart tissue, and these changes outline the organ's structure. Nuclear magnetic resonance is just starting to be used to investigate diseases of heart structure.

One of the most exciting developments in cardiology over the past five years has been balloon angioplasty (see figure 23). In this technique, a catheter with a balloon on its tip is advanced across a tight valve or narrowed blood vessel and inflated, thereby opening the constricted area. Lasers, which are powerful and narrowly focused light beams, are being employed in cardiac surgery on an experimental basis.

Heart transplantation is far and away the most dramatic cardiac surgery, although relatively few transplants have been performed in children. All have been done as a last recourse in patients whose hearts were failing, usually from cardiomyopathy. Heart transplantation in infants and children raises many important questions: what effect will post-transplant medication have on the child's ability to grow? Will the transplanted heart function adequately while he or she grows? What are the long-term physical and emotional problems associated with heart transplantation? Should public money be used to help cover the enormous costs?

In late 1984, public attention was focused on Loma Linda University Medical Center in California where Baby Fae struggled for twenty-one days with a baboon heart. Baby Fae had been born with a hypoplastic left ventricle (see appendix C). These babies usually do not survive longer than a month. A surgical team led by Dr. Leonard Bailey removed Baby Fae's malformed heart and replaced it with one from a baboon. The operation raised a good deal of controversy, but Bailey showed that cross-species heart transplantation is technically feasible and might serve as a stopgap until a human heart is available. Donor hearts for eligible infants are scarce.

In 1986, the infants known as Baby Jesse and Baby Calvin received new hearts from human donors in widely publicized operations. Such babies face an uncertain future, even though new drugs have been developed that help to ward off rejection of the heart by the infant's immune system. Through 1986, only one infant had survived more than a year with a heart transplant. Clearly, much more needs to be learned about heart transplantation before its promise can be realized.

APPENDIXES

Appendix A
THE HEART
PEOPLE

When your child is evaluated or cared for at a medical center, there are a number of people you will encounter. Sometimes the hierarchy in these centers is difficult to understand. You may become confused by seeking information from too many of the staff at various levels; their answers may differ. It is helpful for you to know the function of each individual and how he or she can help you and your child. Although a number of physicians and members of a surgical and cardiac team may be involved in the care of your child, only one physician is ultimately responsible. Talk directly with him or her. Wait for the cardiologist, surgeon, or senior fellow on the service to make rounds so you can get information, rather than trying to piece it together from different sources.

The Medical and Hospital Staff

Cardiologists. Cardiologists are physicians who have special training in diseases of the heart and blood vessels. The field of cardiology is divided into two areas: adult cardiology, which is primarily concerned with the problems adults have with their cardiovascular system, and pediatric cardiology, which is concerned with diseases of newborns, infants, children, and adolescents. Adult and pediatric cardiolgists have different interests, expertise, and training.

An individual who specializes in pediatric cardiology has special training. Following completion of medical school, he or she must have three years of training in general pediatrics to qualify as a pediatrician, a specialist in diseases of children. This is followed by three to four years of training that deals only with diseases of the heart and circulation. At this time, the doctor is eligible for a special examination, which, if successfully completed, entitles the candidate to receive his or her Boards in pediatric cardiology. Currently, there are only about six hundred Board-certified pediatric cardiologists in the United States.

Pediatric cardiologists are responsible for diagnosing the heart problem, perhaps by performing a cardiac catheterization or echocardiogram. They are usually involved in the day-to-day care of the child immediately following an operation. They are also responsible for the long-term postoperative management and follow-up.

Cardiac Surgeons. Cardiac surgeons generally perform surgery on the hearts of both adults and children, but there has been a growing tendency for surgeons to specialize in the care of either children or adults. This is especially true at large university hospitals and children's hospitals.

To become a surgeon, one must go through a long period of training following medical school. A candidate studies general surgery for five to seven years. Following that he or she takes cardiothoracic surgery and training programs lasting from two to three years. During this period the candidate is a resident or fellow in a hospital. Following the completion of this training period, the candidate is eligible to take the board examination in cardiothoracic surgery.

The cardiac surgeon is responsible for patients during hospitalization for surgery. He or she makes the decisions before and after the operation, together with assistance from a pediatric cardiologist. During the operation, the surgeon is responsible for all events that take place in the operating room. If there is a complication following the operation that is directly related to the surgery, the cardiac surgeon is responsible for correcting it.

At most large medical centers, decisions regarding the care and management of the patients are made at conferences in which cardiologists, surgeons, and perhaps other physicians such as anesthesiologists or cardiac radiologists meet, review the patients' films, discuss their situations, and make recommendations concerning their care.

Most cardiac surgery on children is performed in teaching hospitals, either university or children's hospitals. These institutions have a responsibility for training medical students, residents, or other physicians specializing in cardiology, surgery, or other areas. They will be actively involved in the care of your child. The cardiologist and surgeon may share their responsibility or delegate responsibility to other doctors or students. The degree of responsibility that is delegated is directly related to the level of their training and expertise.

The trainees include medical students, interns, residents, and fellows.

Medical Students. Sometimes called student doctors, medical students are not physicians but are in medical school studying to become M.D.'s. They are an important part of the group caring for your child. By meeting and talking with you after examining your child, they are learning the skills that will be essential to them once they are doctors themselves. You can help them learn these skills.

Interns. Interns are doctors who have just graduated from medical school and are in their first year of practical training. They are directly involved in the day-to-day care of your child.

Residents. Residents are physicians who are still in training but have been working in the hospital for several years. Residents supervise the activities of medical students and interns and are important teachers for them. They are responsible for seeing that the medications, examinations, and treatments are properly and efficiently carried out.

Fellows. Fellows are physicians who are studying in great detail a medical subspecialty such as pediatric cardiology or cardiac surgery. They are well-trained individuals who work in a master-apprentice relationship with cardiologists or surgeons to learn the field. Under supervision, they help perform many procedures such as echocardiography, cardiac catheterization, or cardiac surgery.

Consultants. Before or after the operation, unexpected problems may arise such as infection or blood or kidney malfunctions. These problems require special knowledge and care. In such cases, your cardiologist or surgeon will seek consultation from experts in these areas. Consultants will examine your child, take an appropriate history, perhaps order some laboratory tests to help them define the problem, and make recommendations. The recommendations are made to the cardiologist or surgeon who then makes decisions in terms of the overall management of your child. Special problems may arise that require the ongoing support and help of a consultant. In these situations, part of your child's care may be delegated to the consultant.

Nurse Clinicians. This is a new role for nurses, which has been developed and incorporated into the care of cardiac patients within the past few years. A nurse clinician has special interest and training in pediatric cardiology. He or she is part of the cardiology staff and helps with patient education, follow-up, communication, and care. The exact role of the nurse clinician may vary from center to center. You might ask if the center where your child is being treated has a nurse clinician. In certain centers, if there is not a nurse clinician, there may be a social worker who is actively involved in the program.

Registered Nurses (RN). Registered nurses are graduates of accredited nursing schools. Most have a three- or four-year nursing degree and many have taken continuing nursing education courses and seminars focusing on heart problems in children. These RN's develop special skills to deal with problems in pediatric cardiology. They administer treatments and medications and help coordinate care. They also make careful observations of your child's condition and communicate changes to physicians.

Licensed Practical Nurses (LPN). Licensed practical nurses usually have a two-year nursing degree and are under the supervision of a registered nurse.

Nursing Assistants. Nursing assistants, aids, and orderlies have received training while working in the hospital. They help the nursing staff by transporting patients and doing many other tasks on the wards or in the clinic.

Dieticians. Dieticians are trained in nutrition and designing diets that are needed to meet special requirements. In newborns or infants with heart disease, special precautions must be taken in preparing formula or other foods, and the dietician helps with these decisions.

Technologists. Technologists are trained in approved schools to help doctors in their efforts to find and treat your child's problem. Medical technologists perform the chemical and microscopic tests in the laboratory. Radiologic technologists perform X-ray studies. If you have questions about what they are doing in your child's case, do not hesitate to ask them.

Station Secretaries. These people work at the central nursing station desk. The secretary is responsible for coordinating activities. He or she schedules tests, receives laboratory test results, pages doctors, and handles miscellaneous paperwork, among other things.

Social Workers. Social workers will help you with any family or financial problems related to the hospital stay. Feel free to ask them for help in these or other matters. They work closely with the medical and nursing staff to be sure that personal needs are met.

Chaplains. Most hospitals have a full-time chaplain available to provide pastoral care to patients and their families.

Appendix B
QUALITY OF CARE AND PATIENT RIGHTS

If your child is one of the nearly forty million Americans hospitalized each year, how will you know if he or she is getting good care? Are the doctors following proper guidelines in prescribing treatment for your child?

Hospitals generally have a number of committees that review the quality of care dispensed. Special and separate committees review all operations and their results: problems with anesthesia, if any; use of blood; and the credentials, capabilities, and training of physicians. In addition, various government and private agencies review hospital procedures and standards on a regular basis.

If you have questions about procedures, recommendations, or actions, you should first ask your doctor. He or she is willing to discuss these matters with you so that you feel comfortable about the care your child is receiving.

Patient Representatives

Many hospitals have a patient relations department whose responsibility is to provide information and to act as personal representatives for patients and their families.

According to a recent report, there are now more than three thousand patient representatives in the nation's hospitals. Most are salaried employees of the hospital and some receive assistance from volunteers. Their job is to cut through red tape in providing service to patients and to handle complaints. They also try to improve communication between patients and doctors. They work closely with the medical and hospital staffs to ensure that each patient's hospital stay is as comfortable as possible.

Second Opinions

If you question the recommendations or plan of your physician, you can ask for a second opinion from another physician. Do not be afraid to tell your doctor that you would like another equally trained and qualified physician to review the case and give a recommendation. When a parent makes such a request, pediatric cardiologists and surgeons are generally cooperative and will send test results and other information to another physician of your choice.

The physician asked to give the second opinion often wants to review the previous studies and may want to examine your child. Your doctor may also ask a colleague to look at your child and discuss the details. Often the cardiologist will send X-rays and information about a particular patient to a colleague with a specialized area of interest that applies to the case. Cardiologists want to have the most current knowledge and expertise available so that they can give the best possible care.

Patient Rights

You and your child have certain rights. In 1972, the Patient's Bill of Rights was established by the American Hospital Association. It addresses these concerns. Today some states require that a bill of rights for patients be posted in all hospitals. It is up to you to see that they are observed. A patient representative can assist you. These rights usually include:

The right to privacy. In a busy hospital, some hospital staff members from time to time may overlook your privacy. For instance, you may be observed by a number of doctors, nurses, and medical students. Ask them to include you in their discussion of your situation. You should expect to be interviewed in a location that allows as much privacy as possible. When your child is being examined, the bedside curtain or door should be closed.

The right to confidentiality. This is a very special right to privacy in which the doctor promises to protect information obtained during the examination or private consultation with you. Your child's hospital record, laboratory reports, or X-rays cannot be sent to others unless you give permission, or unless the hospital is compelled to do so by a court order or special regulation.

The right to understand. You have a right to have the nature of your child's heart problem and the recommended treatment explained to you in terms that you understand. The reason for the treatment, its potential benefits and risks, and alternatives should be made clear to you. Often doctors use medical terms that you may not comprehend. Ask them to provide a simpler explanation.

The right to consent or refuse. For operations, cardiac catheterizations, or other major procedures, your written consent will be requested. Before signing the consent form, you should fully understand the nature, risks, and benefits of the procedure. Your doctor will explain them to you. Be sure to ask if you do not understand them.

Your Responsibilities as Parents

To be honest. Give a reliable history of your child's illness.

To try to understand. Make an effort to learn about your child's disease and the way it is being treated. This is very important for successful treatment.

To report changes in your child's health. Even seemingly insignificant changes could be important.

To keep your child's medical appointments.

To follow the treatment plan. Know what medications are being prescribed for your child and how often they should be administered.

To acquaint yourself with the medical staff. You will be more likely to ask questions and have your concerns addressed if you are acquainted with the staff.

To be considerate. If your child shares a hospital room, allow the other patient his or her privacy. Limit visitors and help maintain a quiet atmosphere.

Appendix C
OTHER KINDS OF CONGENITAL HEART DISEASE

Patent Ductus Arteriosus

The ductus arteriosus is a connection between the aorta and pulmonary artery (fig. 27). This connection is present in every fetus and generally closes within 48 hours of birth. If for some reason it remains open, however, the result is patent ductus arteriosus. This causes some of the oxygen-rich blood to flow from the aorta back through the lungs, thus escaping the normal route of circulation.

In many infants with this condition, the circumference of the ductus is very small, allowing little blood to recirculate wastefully. Those babies that have a large ductus may develop pneumonia and tire easily. They may also develop congestive heart failure. Patent ductus arteriosus is easily corrected by surgery, and the recovery period is generally brief.

Patent ductus arteriosus is common in premature infants and also tends to be more frequent in smaller babies, particularly those under one thousand grams (approximately two pounds). The presence of this condition may complicate respiratory problems that often beset these babies. Medications are proving to be effective in closing the ductus arteriosus in premature infants.

Atrial Septal Defect

An atrial septal defect is a hole in the septum (wall) that separates the left from the right atrium (fig. 28). Because the pressure is higher in the left atrium, blood flows through the defect from the left to the right atrium and recirculates through the lungs.

Most of these defects are large and permit free blood flow through the

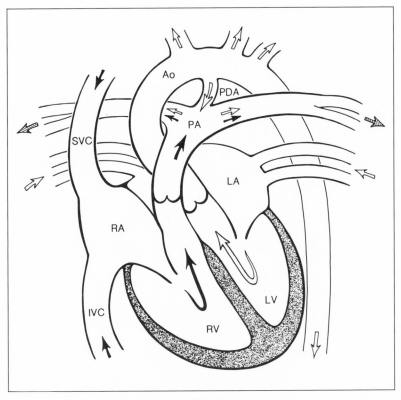

FIGURE 27

Patent ductus arteriosus. In this anomaly a connection (PDA) exists between the aorta (Ao) and pulmonary artery (PA). Because the pressure in
the aorta is higher than in the PA, blood flows from the aorta through the
PDA into the PA, and, therefore, oxygen-rich blood flows through the
lungs. Thus there is excess volume of blood through the lungs. (SVC = superior vena cava, IVC = inferior vena cava, RA = right atrium, RV = right
ventricle, LA = left atrium, LV = left ventricle)

right side of the heart. The right atrium and ventricle are well equipped to
handle this excessive blood volume, so most patients show no symptoms
of the problem through childhood. As they mature, however, the prolonged effect of excessive blood flow through the lungs begins to have an
effect. The blood vessels in the lungs narrow and raise the pressure on the
right side of the heart. Symptoms develop during the third, fourth, or fifth
decades of life.

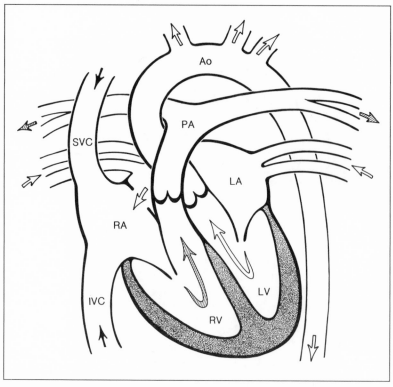

FIGURE 28

Atrial septal defect. In this anomaly a defect is present in the wall between the left atrium (LA) and the right atrium (RA). Because the pressure is higher in the LA than in the RA, oxygen-rich blood flows through the defect. Therefore, extra blood flows through the chambers of the right side of the heart and lungs. (SVC = superior vena cava, IVC = inferior vena cava, Ao = aorta, PA = pulmonary artery, RV = right ventricle, LV = left ventricle)

Atrial septal defect is often detected by the discovery of a murmur in a preschool physical examination. Before that, the condition is difficult to diagnose because the murmur is similar to a normal murmur.

Surgery during childhood can prevent long-term consequences, and the risk is low. Often a cardiac catheterization is not necessary before the operation because the diagnosis can be made with an echocardiogram and clinical evaluation.

Endocardial Cushion Defect

Endocardial cushion defect encompasses a spectrum of congenital heart defects that involve the endocardial cushions, two structures of the early developing heart. The endocardial cushions are extremely important in heart formation because they contribute to the development of the atrial and ventricular septa and the mitral and tricuspid valves. All four of these critical structures can be affected in infants with the defect.

The most common form of endocardial cushion defect involves the atrial septum and the mitral valve (ostium primum defect with cleft mitral valve) (fig. 29). A leak in the mitral valve causes some blood to flow in the wrong direction, back into the left atrium through the defective valve. Mild regurgitation is usually well tolerated, but severe disease places great stress on the left side of the heart and can cause congestive heart failure. In a few patients, symptoms of heart failure develop in infancy.

Heart failure in infants is more common in another form of endocardial cushion defect that involves the atrial and ventricular septa and the mitral and tricuspid valves (complete atrioventricular canal). In both forms a murmur is the first clue. The diagnosis is generally made with the electro- and echocardiogram because characteristic features are almost always present. Usually catheterization is performed to confirm the diagnosis.

Surgical repair of these defects is difficult because of the delicate tissues involved. In newborns with severe disease, such repair is associated with high operative risk. At some centers a temporizing procedure is performed that reduces the load on the heart. Later on, when the infant is better able to tolerate it, corrective surgery is done. Afterward some mitral valve leakage may continue, but usually this is well tolerated.

Pulmonary Stenosis

Like aortic stenosis (see chapter 4), pulmonary stenosis obstructs blood flow from the heart, but on the right side rather than the left (fig. 30). Pressure is increased in the right ventricle and the ventricular wall thickens in response to the obstruction.

The obstruction can be so severe that the right ventricle cannot generate sufficient pressure to deliver an adequate flow of blood to the lungs. The child develops features of congestive cardiac failure. In other instances, the pressure on the atrial septum prevents the fetal passageway from closing after birth. As a result, blood flows from the right into the left atrium, and the child becomes cyanotic.

Again, a murmur is usually the first diagnostic clue. Usually the murmur is loud and can be heard in the neonatal period. Echocardiography is done to evaluate the severity of the obstruction, often followed by catheteriza-

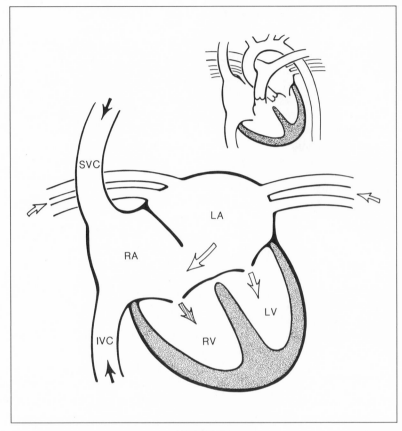

FIGURE 29

Endocardial cushion defect. (Also called AV canal or ostium primum defect.) In the large diagram the pulmonary artery and aorta have been removed for easier presentation. In this anomaly there is a communication
between the left atrium (LA) and the right atrium (RA). In addition, there
is a communication between the left ventricle (LV) and the right ventricle
(RV). In some cases a common valve between the atrium and the ventricles
as well. (SVC = superior vena cava, IVC = inferior vena cava)

tion, at which time a balloon may be inflated in the narrowed valve to open
it. At other times an operation is performed to open the valve. Infants with
a mild degree of obstruction may not require surgery at all, but those with
cyanosis, heart failure, or other signs of severe stenosis undergo a pulmonary valvotomy: the narrowed valve is surgically widened, often by the use

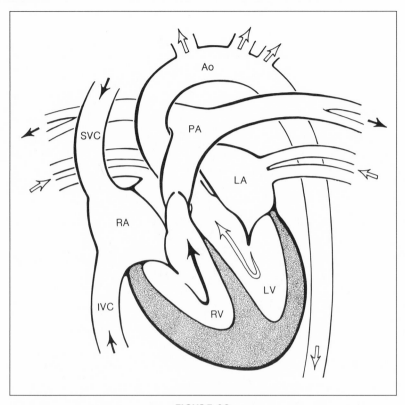

FIGURE 30

Pulmonary stenosis. In this condition the pulmonary valve that separates the right ventricle (RV) from the pulmonary artery (PA) is narrowed and does not open fully. As a result, the pressure in the RV increases. (SVC = superior vena cava, IVC = inferior vena cava, RA = right atrium, Ao = aorta, LA = left atrium, LV = left ventricle)

of a patch. Following this operation, the pulmonary valve may continue to leak and the murmur may persist, but infants can usually tolerate this well.

Coarctation of the Aorta

Coarctation or narrowing of the aorta is a fairly common cardiac anomaly (fig. 31). Blood pressure in the aorta is elevated above the constriction

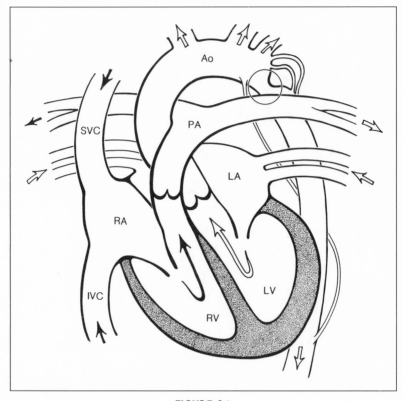

FIGURE 31

Coarctation of the aorta. In this condition there is a narrowing in the aorta (Ao) (shown within the circle). Because of this narrowing, the pressure in the aorta and left ventricle (LV) increases. To help carry blood from the portion of the aorta before the obstruction to that beyond, blood vessels enlarge around it. Three of these blood vessels are indicated in this diagram. (SVC = superior vena cava, IVC = inferior vena cava, RA = right atrium, PA = pulmonary artery, RV = right ventricle, LA = left atrium)

and normal or decreased below it. Indeed, high blood pressure is often the first clue. Although many people who have the condition are diagnosed later in life, some infants have a severe constriction leading to cardiac failure.

Diagnosis of coarctation of the aorta is usually made by the discovery of high blood pressure in the arms and lower pressure in the legs. (These

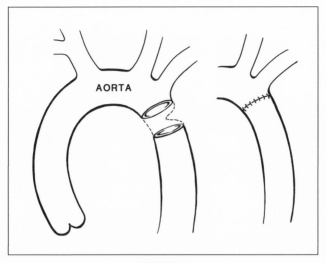

FIGURE 32

End-to-end anastomosis. This is an operation for coarctation of the aorta. The narrowed segment of the aorta is removed, and the ends of the aorta are sewn together.

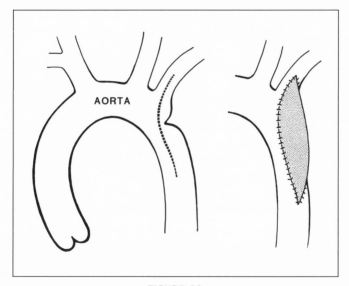

FIGURE 33

Patch angioplasty. This is an operation for coarctation of the aorta. **Left:** An incision is made in the aorta and into the blood vessel going to the left arm. **Right:** A piece of synthetic material is sewn into the incision.

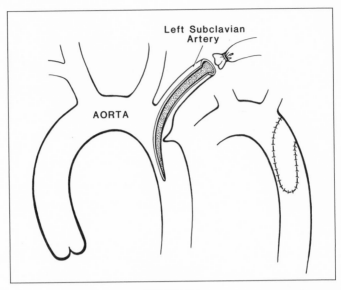

FIGURE 34

Subclavian flap. This is an operation for coarctation of the aorta. **Left:** The left subclavian artery is divided and then opened along its course and on into the aorta, across the narrowed area. **Right:** The subclavian artery is then turned down into the aorta, across the coarctation site, and sewn to widen this narrowed area.

pressures are normally equal.) Heart murmurs may also be present. X-rays and echocardiogram are very helpful in making the diagnosis and identifying the site of the coarctation.

Most children with coarctation of the aorta require an operation. In severely affected infants, it is an emergency procedure; in milder cases surgery may be elective or recommended before the child begins school. The operation involves removing the constricted segment and sewing the aorta back together (fig. 32). Sometimes a patch of synthetic material is used to widen the constriction (fig. 33); at other times the major artery to the arm is divided, opened, and used as a flap to widen the constriction (fig. 34). Long-term follow-up is necessary because some patients may have hypertension. About half the patients with the condition have an aortic valve with two instead of the normal three cusps. Occasionally the obstruction recurs and a second operation is necessary.

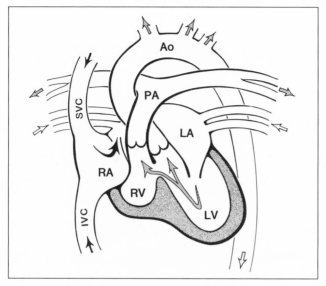

FIGURE 35

Tricuspid atresia. The tricuspid valve is sealed closed. Thus the blood returning from the body cannot enter the right ventricle (RV), so it flows from the right atrium (RA) to the left atrium (LA). From the LA, the blood flows into the left ventricle (LV). Blood from the LV is pumped into the aorta (Ao), and through a ventricular septal defect, into the pulmonary artery (PA). (SVC = superior vena cava, IVC = inferior vena cava)

Tricuspid Atresia

The tricuspid valve permits blood to flow from the right atrium into the right ventricle (fig. 35). In tricuspid atresia this valve is absent, and blood passes through a defect in the atrial septum from the right atrium to the left atrium where it mixes with blood returning from the lungs. This mixture, in turn, flows into the left ventricle, where a portion is pumped into the aorta and another portion into the pulmonary artery through a ventricular septal defect.

Infants with tricuspid atresia are often cyanotic and require some form of surgery early in life. Although this congenital disease is generally diagnosed by electrocardiographic and echocardiographic findings, catheterization is done to confirm the diagnosis, define the size of the ventricular septal defect, and measure the outflow to the lungs. Catheterization is also used to perform a balloon atrial septostomy, which allows blood to exit freely from the right atrium. In newborns, a shunt procedure may be

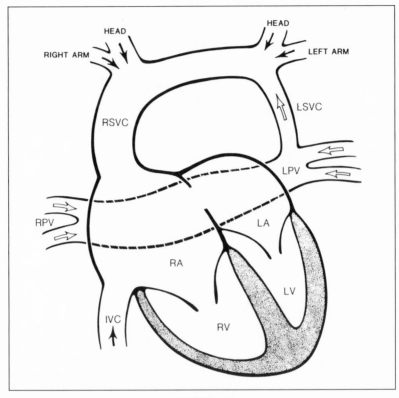

FIGURE 36

A type of total anomalous pulmonary venous connection. In this diagram the pulmonary artery and aorta have been removed for easier presentation. The pulmonary veins from the right lung (RPV) and from the left lung (LPV) do not join the left atrium (LA) as usual. Instead they join a blood vessel called the left superior vena cava (LSVC), which then joins blood vessels from the arms and head to flow into the right superior vena cava (RSVC) and into the right atrium (RA). Thus all the blood returning to the heart enters the RA. From the RA blood flows normally into the right ventricle (RV) and also through a hole in the atrial septum into the LA. (IVC = inferior vena cava, LV = left ventricle)

needed to improve blood flow to the lungs and to prevent cyanosis. In children who are at least two years old, a procedure that connects the right atrium to the right ventricle or pulmonary artery, called a Fontan procedure, is sometimes done.

Despite improvements in diagnosis and surgery, tricuspid atresia remains a serious defect. Long-term results of treatment are being evaluated.

Total Anomalous Pulmonary Venous Connection

Infants with total anomalous pulmonary venous connection have pulmonary veins that do not connect to the left atrium (fig. 36), a connection that normally occurs during early heart development in the fetus. As a result, these vessels form an abnormal vascular connection to the right atrium. All blood returning to the heart, from the lungs as well as the body, is delivered to the right atrium, where a portion flows into the right ventricle and lungs and another portion passes through an atrial septal defect into the left side of the heart and then into the body.

Most patients have a markedly increased blood flow through the lungs. Children with the condition show symptoms in infancy, such as congestive heart failure, and are often beset by respiratory infections, including pneumonia. Infants in whom the abnormal connecting channel is constricted are cyanotic and require surgery immediately. An opening is made in the back wall of the left atrium, and the junction of the pulmonary veins is connected to this opening. The connecting vein is divided and the atrial septal defect is closed. Operations on newborns with an obstruction carry a higher risk than those on older infants who do not have an obstructed vessel.

Ebstein's Malformation

In Ebstein's malformation, the tricuspid valve is located within the right ventricle rather than at the junction of the right atrium and right ventricle (fig. 37). This results in an enlarged right atrium and a smaller right ventricle (the pumping chamber). An atrial septal defect that allows blood to flow from the right into the left atrium is also present.

In some cases, affected newborns are cyanotic and may have congestive heart failure, although these conditions may gradually improve. For babies with no improvement, an operative technique has been developed in which the tricuspid valve is replaced or repaired and the atrial septal defect is closed. Surgery relieves symptoms, but the long-term outlook for valvular replacements is not known.

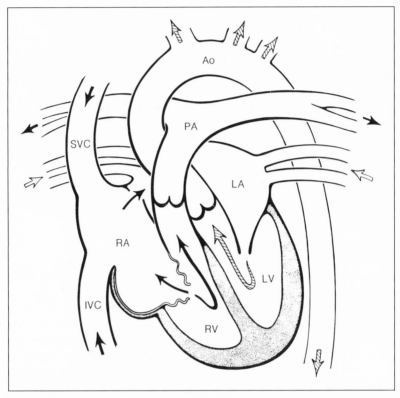

FIGURE 37

Ebstein's malformation of tricuspid valve. The tricuspid valve is displaced into the right ventricle (RV). This valve is insufficient and allows blood to regurgitate into the right atrium (RA). Blood from the inferior vena cava (IVC) and superior vena cava (SVC) flows into the RV and also through an atrial communication into the left atrium (LA). (Ao = aorta, PA = pulmonary artery, LV = left ventricle)

Hypoplastic Left Ventricle

Hypoplastic left ventricle applies to a spectrum of defects involving the aortic or mitral valves in which the left ventricle is too small to support life (fig. 38). One or both valves may be sealed shut or severely narrowed so that blood flow through the left side of the heart is constricted or cut off. Circulation depends solely on the pumping action of the right ventricle. When the

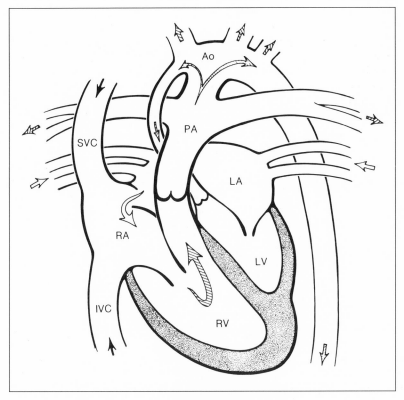

FIGURE 38

Hypoplastic left ventricle with aortic atresia. The aortic valve is atretic so no blood flows from the hypoplastic (small) left ventricle (LV) to the aorta (Ao). Blood returns to the right atrium (RA) from the inferior vena cava (IVC) and the superior vena cava (SVC). This blood enters the right ventricle (RV) and is pumped into the pulmonary artery (PA). Most of this blood flows into the aorta through a patent ductus arteriosus. Blood returning to the left atrium (LA) from the lungs passes through an atrial communication to the RA.

ductus arteriosus closes during the first days following birth, the major source of blood for the body in affected newborns is progressively reduced.

Symptoms include breathing difficulty, a mottled appearance, poor pulse, and low blood pressure. Congestive heart failure is often present. Physicians can usually make a diagnosis with the help of an echocardiogram. At some centers, cardiac catheterization and angiography are also done.

Unlike the outlook for patients with other congenital heart defects, infants with hypoplastic left ventricle usually do not live longer than a month after birth. An experimental operation has not significantly improved the outlook for these babies and most cardiologists do not recommend it. However, as surgeons become more experienced in dealing with the defect, perhaps this operation will one day offer hope.

Appendix D
PROFESSIONAL ASSOCIATIONS AND PARENT SUPPORT GROUPS

The American Heart Association

The American Heart Association was founded in 1924 by six New York City cardiologists. Currently it has active organizations in all fifty states and Puerto Rico (addresses and telephone numbers are listed below) and components in more than one thousand communities, making it one of the world's largest voluntary health organizations. The AHA raises millions of dollars for research each year and sponsors programs for public education, professional development, and community service in the fight against heart and blood vessel diseases, the nation's number one killer.

United States

American Heart Association
National Center
7320 Greenville Avenue
Dallas, TX 75231
214/750-5300

Alabama Affiliate
P.O. Box 9097
Birmingham, AL 35213
205/592-7100

Alaska Affiliate
2330 East 42d Street
Anchorage, AK 99504
907/563-3111

Arizona Affiliate
1445 East Thomas
Phoenix, AZ 85014
602/277-4846

Arkansas Affiliate
P.O. Box 1610
Little Rock, AR 72203
501/375-9148

California Affiliate
805 Burlway Road
Burlingame, CA 94010
415/342-5522

Chicago Heart Association
20 N. Wacker Drive
Chicago, IL 60606
312/346-4675

Colorado Heart Association
P.O. Box 22066
Denver, CO 80222
303/399-2131

Connecticut Affiliate, Inc.
71 Parker Avenue
Meriden, CT 06450
203/634-4532

Dakota Affiliate
P.O. Box 1287
Jamestown, ND 58401
701/252-5122

American Heart Association of
Delaware, Inc.
4C Trolley Square
Delaware Avenue and
  DuPont Street
Wilmington, DE 19806
302/654-5269

Nation's Capital Affiliate
(District of Columbia)
2233 Wisconsin Avenue N.W.
Washington, D.C. 20007
202/337-6400

Florida Affiliate
P.O. Box 42150
St. Petersburg, FL 33742
813/522-9477

Georgia Affiliate
P.O. Box 13589
Atlanta, GA 30324
404/261-2260

American Heart Association
Hawaii, Inc.
245 North Kukui Street
Honolulu, HI 96817
808/538-7021

American Heart Association of
Idaho, Inc.
3295 Elder Street, Suite 140
Boise, ID 83705
208/384-5066

Illinois Affiliate
P.O. Box 2666
Springfield, IL 62708
217/525-1350

Indiana Affiliate, Inc.
222 S. Downey, Suite 222
Indianapolis, IN 46219
317/357-8622

Iowa Affiliate
1111 Office Park Road
West Des Moines, IA 50265
515/224-1025

Kansas Affiliate
5229 West 7th Street
Topeka, KA 66606
913/272-7056

Kentucky Affiliate, Inc.
207 Speed Building
Louisville, KY 40202
502/587-8641

Greater Los Angeles Affiliate
2405 West 8th Street
Los Angeles, CA 90057
213/385-4231

Louisiana, Inc.
P.O. Box 19122
New Orleans, LA 70179
504/827-1644

Maine Affiliate, Inc.
20 Winter Street
August, ME 04330
207/623-8432

Maryland Affiliate, Inc.
P.O. Box 17025
Baltimore, MD 21203
301/685-7074

Massachusetts Affiliate, Inc.
33 Fourth Avenue
Needham Heights, MA 02194
617/449-5931

AHA of Michigan
P.O. Box 160-LV
Lathrup Village, MI 48076
313/557-9500

Minnesota Affiliate, Inc.
4701 West 77th Street
Minneapolis, MN 55435
612/835-3300

Mississippi Affiliate
P.O. Box 16063
Jackson, MS 39236
601/981-4721

Missouri Affiliate
P.O. Box Q
Columbia, MO 65201
314/442-3193

Montana Affiliate
510 1st Avenue N.
Great Falls, MT 59401
406/452-2362

Nebraska Affiliate
3624 Farnam
Omaha, NE 68131
402/346-0771

Nevada Affiliate
1135 Terminal Way
Suites 104 and 105
Reno, NV 89502
702/322-2977

New Hampshire Affiliate
RFD #4, Box 337-B
Concord, NH 03301
603/224-7461

New Jersey Affiliate
1525 Morris Avenue
Union, NJ 07083
201/688-4540

New Mexico Affiliate
2403 San Mateo, N.E.
Suite W-14
Albuquerque, NM 87110
505/884-3717

New York State Affiliate
214 South Warren Street
Syracuse, NY 13202
315/478-6681

New York Heart Association
205 East 42d Street
New York, N.Y. 10017
212/661-5335

North Carolina Affiliate
P.O. Box 2636
Chapel Hill, NC 27514
919/968-4453

Northeast Ohio Affiliate
1689 East 115th Street
Cleveland, OH 44106
216/791-7500

Ohio Affiliate, Inc.
6161 Busch Boulevard, Suite 327
Columbus, OH 43229
614/436-0958

Oklahoma Affiliate, Inc.
P.O. Box 11376
Oklahoma City, OK 73136
405/521-9838

Oregon Affiliate
1500 S.W. 12th Avenue
Portland, OR 97201
503/226-2575

Pennsylvania Affiliate
P.O. Box 2435
Harrisburg, PA 17105
717/238-0895

Puerto Rico Heart Association
Cabo Alverio 554
Hato Rey
Puerto Rico 00918
809/763-8275

Rhode Island Affiliate
40 Broad Street
Pawtucket, RI 02860
401/728-5300

South Carolina Affiliate
P.O. Box 6604
Columbia, SC 29203
803/738-9540

Tennessee Affiliate
101 23d Avenue
Nashville, TN 37203
615/320-0390

Texas Affiliate, Inc.
P.O. Box 15186
Austin, TX 78761
512/836-7220

Utah Heart Association
645E-400S
Salt Lake City, UT 84102
801/322-5601

Vermont Affiliate, Inc.
R.D. #2, Box 2821
Shelburne, VT 05482
802/985-8048

Virginia Affiliate, Inc.
4217 Park Place Court
Glen Valley, VA 23060
804/747-8334

AHA of Washington
4414 Woodland Park Avenue N.
Seattle, WA 98103
206/632-6881

West Virginia Affiliate
211 35th Street S.E.
Charleston, WV 25304
304/346-5381

Wisconsin Affiliate, Inc.
795 North Van Buren Street
Milwaukee, WI 53202
414/271-9999

AHA of Wyoming, Inc.
2015 Central Avenue
Cheyenne, WY 82001
307/632-1746

Canada

Ontario Heart Foundation
247 Davenport Road
Toronto 180, Ontario

Nova Scotia Heart Foundation
P.O. Box 1585
406 Roy Building
Halifax, N.S.

Manitoba Heart Foundation
313 Canada Building
352 Donald Street
Winnipeg 2, Manitoba

Saskatchewan Heart Foundation
708 Canada Building
105 21st Street East
Saskatoon, Saskatchewan

Alberta Heart Foundation
2011 10th Avenue S.W.
Calgary 4, Alberta

Alberta Heart Foundation
10102 101st Street
Edmonton 15, Alberta

Quebec Heart Foundation
Fondation Du Quebec
Des Maladies Du Coeur
1455 Rue Peel Street
Suite M−31/31
Montreal 110, Quebec

Canadian Heart Foundation
New Brunswick Division
28 Germain Street
Saint John
New Brunswick

Canadian Heart Foundation
Newfoundland Division
Avalon Mall
St. John's
Newfoundland

Canadian Heart Foundation
Prince Edward Island Division
P.O. Box 279
Charlottetown, P.E.I.

British Columbia
Heart Foundation
1881 West Broadway
Vancouver 9, B.C.

United Kingdom

British Heart Foundation
57 Gloucester Place
London, WIH 4DH

Regional Offices

Northumberland, Cumbria, Durham, Tyne, Wear, and Cleveland

British Heart Foundation
393 Westgate Road
Newcastle upon Tyne, NE4 6PA

Norfolk, Suffolk, Cambridgeshire, Herts, Beds, Bucks, Essex, and Northants

British Heart Foundation
1 Market Street
Saffron Walden
Essex, CB10 1HZ

Scotland

British Heart Foundation
16 Chester Street
Edinburgh, EH3 7RA

London—Northern, Southern, and Eastern Boroughs

British Heart Foundation
Langthorne Hospital
Langthorne Road
London, E11 4HJ

Lancashire, Merseyside, Cheshire, Greater Manchester, and Northern Ireland

British Heart Foundation
5 Castle Street
Liverpool, L2 4SW

Kent, Surrey, East and West Sussex, Hampshire, Berkshire, and Isle of Wight

British Heart Foundation
33 High Street
Ticehurst
Wadhurst
East Sussex, TN5 7AS

Glos, Avon, Oxon, Dorest, Somerset, Wilts, Devon, and Cornwall

British Heart Foundation
6 Terrace Walk
Bath
Avon, BA1 1LN

Leicestershire, Derbyshire, Lincolnshire, Notts, South Humberside, West Midlands, Warwickshire, and Staffordshire

British Heart Foundation
32 Park Row
Nottingham, NG1 6GR

Yorkshire and North Humberside

British Heart Foundation
93a Albion Street
Leeds, LS1 5AP

London—Western Boroughs

British Heart Foundation
29 Walham Grove
London, SW6 1QR

Wales, Shropshire, Hereford, and Worcester

British Heart Foundation
Brighton House
Temple Street
Llandrindod Wells
Powys, LD1 5DH

Parent Support Groups

Support groups for parents of children with cardiovascular disease enable
you to share your experiences and to learn about your child's special needs.

Parents for Heart of Minnesota
2525 Chicago Avenue S.
Minneapolis, MN 55404

Parents for Heart
Chicago Heart Association,
Rm. 240
20 North Wacker Drive
Chicago, IL 60606

Parents for Heart
2631 11th Avenue N.W.
Rochester, MN 55901

Parents for Heart
618 South 14th Street
Fargo, ND 58103

Parents of Cardiac Children
of Children United
386 Main Street
Middletown, CT 06457

Hearts for Children
2309 Albright Drive
Greensboro, NC 27408

Parents for Heart
4310 Glenwood
Duluth, MN 55804

Congenital Heart Information
Program
P.O. Box 15131
Baton Rouge, LA 70895

Appendix E
PROGRAM FOR PREVENTION OF ATHEROSCLEROSIS

Your efforts to develop healthy habits in your children can pay off by a decreased likelihood of heart attack and stroke in their adult years. The program aimed at prevention should include:

1. Development of eating habits that will promote a diet with an adequate, but not excessive, amount of calories, fat, cholesterol, and salt. Such a diet should include: cholesterol, less than three hundred milligrams per day; total calories from fat, less than 30 percent; total calories from saturated fat, less than 10 percent; and salt, no more than five grams per day.

2. Prevention or treatment of obesity.

3. Prevention of smoking.

4. Physical activity and regular exercise.

5. Identification and management of children with hypertension or high blood pressure and those with hypercholesterolemia or a high level of cholesterol in their blood. These children often have a family history of high blood pressure or high cholesterol.

Such a program for your family is inexpensive and easy to carry out but requires you to modify your habits as well. It cannot be said too often that children's habits are developed early in life and are influenced primarily by the habits and attitudes of their parents.

Currently a number of government and voluntary health agencies are directing educational programs toward modifying risk factors in adults, and these programs should also benefit children, at least indirectly, by helping to change the habits of their parents that contribute to heart disease.

SUGGESTED
READINGS

SUGGESTED READINGS

1986 Heart Facts, American Heart Association (hereafter AHA), item no. 55–005J.

Abnormalities of Heart Rhythm – A guide for Parents, AHA, item no. 50–058A.

About High Blood Pressure in Children – What Parents Should Know, AHA, item no. 50–045A.

About Your Heart and Diet, AHA, item no. 51–040A.

About Your Heart and Exercise, AHA, item no. 51–038A.

About Your Heart and Smoking, AHA, item no. 51–037A.

About Your Heart and Bloodstream, AHA, item no. 51–031A.

American Heart Association Diet, AHA, item no. 51–018B.

Children and Smoking – A Message to Parents, AHA, item no. 51–033A.

Cholesterol and Your Heart, AHA, item no. 50–069A.

Dental Care of Children with Heart Disease, AHA, item no. 50–043A.

Dr. Truso's Jet Powered Pedaler Comic Book, AHA, item no. 64–009J.

Facts About Congestive Heart Failure, AHA, item no. 51–007A.

Feeding Infants with Congenital Heart Diseases – A Guide for Parents, AHA, item no. 50–070A.

If Your Child Has a Congenital Heart Defect, AHA, item no. 50–014B.

Innocent Heart Murmurs in Children, AHA, item no. 51–014C.

Putting Your Heart Into Curriculum, Primary Level-Kindergarten-2nd Grade, AHA, item no. 95–020B.

Putting Your Heart Into Curriculum, Intermediate Level-Grades 3–5, AHA, item no. 95–020C.

Putting Your Heart Into Curriculum, Junior Level-Grades 6–8, AHA, item no. 95–020D.

Putting Your Heart Into Curriculum, Senior Level, AHA, item no. 95–020E.

Road to a Healthy Heart Game, AHA, item no. 56–003A.

Songs from the Heart Songbook, AHA, item no. 64–0090.

Tin Woodsman "Take Care of Your Heart" Activity Book, AHA, item no. 64–009M.

You and Heart Surgery, AHA, item no. CHICAGO HEART.

For additional publications by the AHA, consult the Public Literature Catalog at your AHA affiliate.

The People's Hospital Book, Dr. Ronald Gots and Dr. Arthur Kaufman. New York: Avon, 1981.

Essentials of Pediatric Cardiology, James H. Moller, M.D. (2d ed.). Philadelphia, PA: F. A. Davis Co., 1978. (A paperback written for medical students and practitioners.)

So You're Having an Operation: A Step by Step Guide to Controlling Your Hospital Stay, Karen R. Williams and Janet Stensaas. Englewood Cliffs, NJ: Prentice-Hall, 1985.

GLOSSARY

GLOSSARY

The following terms were selected largely from *1986 Heart Facts,* published by the American Heart Association, 1985. Reprinted with permission.

Aneurysm. A ballooning-out of the wall of a vein, an artery, or the heart owing to weakening of the wall by disease, traumatic injury, or an abnormality present at birth.

Angiocardiography. An X-ray examination of the heart and blood vessels that traces the course of an opaque fluid that has been injected into the bloodstream.

Aorta. The main trunk artery that receives blood from the left ventricle of the heart and distributes it to other arteries.

Arrhythmia (or Dysrhythmia). An abnormal rhythm of the heart.

Arteriosclerosis. Commonly called "hardening of the arteries." It includes a variety of conditions that cause the artery walls to thicken and lose elasticity.

Artery. Any large blood vessel that carries blood from the heart to the various parts of the body.

Atherosclerosis. A form of arteriosclerosis in which the inner layers of artery walls become thick and irregular owing to deposits of a fatty substance. When the interior walls of arteries become lined with layers of these deposits, the arteries become narrowed, and the flow of blood through the arteries is reduced.

Atrium. One of the two upper chambers of the heart in which blood collects before being passed to the ventricles.

Blood Pressure. The force or pressure exerted by the heart in pumping blood; the pressure of blood in the arteries.

"Blue Babies." Babies who have a blue tinge to their skin (cyanosis) resulting from insufficient oxygen in the arterial blood. This often indicates a heart defect.

Capillaries. Very small blood vessels that distribute oxygenated blood to all parts of the body.

Cardiac. Pertaining to the heart.

Cardiac arrest. When the heart stops beating.

Cardiology. The study of the heart and its functions in health and disease.

Cardiovascular. Pertaining to the heart and blood vessels.

Catheterization. The process of examining the heart by introducing a thin tube (catheter) into a vein or artery and passing it into the heart.

Cholesterol. A fatlike substance found only in animal tissue.

Circulatory System. The heart, arteries, veins, and capillaries through which the blood moves as it flows through the body.

Congenital Defects. Malformation of the heart or of its major blood vessels present at birth.

Congestive Heart Failure. The inability of the heart to pump out all the blood that returns to it. This results in the backing up of blood in the veins that lead to the heart and sometimes in the accumulation of fluid in various parts of the body.

Coronary Arteries. Two arteries, arising from the aorta, arching down over the heart, branching, and bringing blood to the heart muscle.

Cyanosis. Blueness of skin caused by insufficient oxygen in the blood.

Defibrillator. An electronic device that helps to reestablish normal contraction rhythms in a heart that is malfunctioning.

Digitalis (also Digoxin, Digitoxin). A drug often used in the treatment of congestive heart failure that strengthens the contraction of the heart and promotes the elimination of fluid from body tissues. It is also sometimes used to treat certain arrhythmias.

Diuretic. A drug that increases the rate of formation of urine by promoting the excretion of water and salts.

Echocardiography. A diagnostic method in which pulses of sound are transmitted into the body and the echoes returning from the surfaces of the heart and other structures are electronically plotted and recorded.

Edema. Swelling that results from abnormally large amounts of fluid in the body tissues.

Electrocardiogram (ECG or EKG). A graphic record of electrical impulses produced by the heart.

Embolus. A blood clot that forms in the blood vessels in one part of the body and is then carried to another part of the body.

Epidemiology. The science dealing with where and how often diseases occur in a human community.

Fibrillation. Uncoordinated contractions of the heart muscle occurring when individual muscle fibers contract on their own.

Heart Attack. A nonspecific term usually referring to a myocardial infarction.

Heart-Lung Machine. An apparatus that oxygenates and pumps blood during open-heart surgery.

High Blood Pressure. An unstable or persistent elevation of blood pressure above the normal range.

Hypertension. High blood pressure.

Myocardial Infarction. The damaging or death of an area of the heart muscle (myocardium) resulting from a reduced blood supply to that area.

Myocardium. The muscular wall of the heart. It contracts to pump blood out of the heart and then relaxes when the heart refills with returning blood.

Obesity. The condition of being significantly overweight. It puts a strain on the heart and increases the chance of developing two major heart attack risk factors—high blood pressure and diabetes.

Open Heart Surgery. Surgery performed on the opened heart while the bloodstream is diverted through a heart-lung machine.

Pacemaker. A small mass of specialized cells in the right atrium of the heart that produces the electrical impulses that cause contractions of the heart. The term artificial pacemaker is applied to an electrical device that can substitute for a defective natural pacemaker and control the beating of the heart by emitting a series of rhythmic electrical discharges.

Platelets. One of three kinds of formed elements found in the blood. It aids in the clotting of blood.

Pulmonary. Pertaining to the lungs.

Rheumatic Heart Disease. Damage done to the heart, particularly to the heart valves, by one or more attacks of rheumatic fever.

Rubella. Commonly known as German measles. A viral illness causing fever and a rash. When a woman develops it during her first three months of pregnancy, the exposed baby may be born with heart disease and other problems.

Septa. The muscular walls dividing the two chambers on the left side of the heart from the two chambers on the right.

Strep Infection (Streptococcal Infection). An infection, usually in the throat, resulting from the presence of the streptococcus bacteria.

Thrombosis. The formation or presence of a blood clot (thrombus) inside a blood vessel or cavity of the heart.

Vascular. Pertaining to the blood vessels.

Vein. Any one of a series of vessels of the vascular system that carries blood from various parts of the body back to the heart.

Ventricle. One of the two lower chambers of the heart.

INDEX

Index

Professor of pediatrics at the University of Minnesota Medical School and chief of staff at the University of Minnesota Hospital and Clinic, **JAMES H. MOLLER,** M.D., has been with the University of Minnesota since 1965. He is active as a health care adviser in the Minneapolis community as well as a member of many professional associations. Moller is on the executive committee of the Minnesota Heart Association and participates in many American Heart Association committees. Widely published, Moller contributes to such journals as *American Journal Diseases of Childhood* and is author of *The Baby Checkup Book* with S. Hillman and R. S. Hillman and *Radiology of Congenital Heart Disease* with K. Amplatz and W. Castañeda-Zuñiga.

WILLIAM A. NEAL, M.D., is a pediatric cardiologist and professor and chairman of pediatric cardiology at the West Virginia University School of Medicine. He was previously a resident and fellow at the University of Minnesota Hospitals. Neal is a member of the Naval Research Advisory Committee and has served as president of the National Perinatal Association. He is coauthor, with Moller, of *Heart Disease in Infancy.*

WILLIAM HOFFMAN is an editor and science writer. In 1976, he received his master's degree in journalism from the University of Minnesota. Hoffman contributes to *Encounters* (published by the Science Museum of Minnesota) and to other local journals.